LUPUS
= Lift Up, Persevere, Use Strength

A Lupus Warrior's Story of Hope, Spirit and Fortitude

Rachel Lea

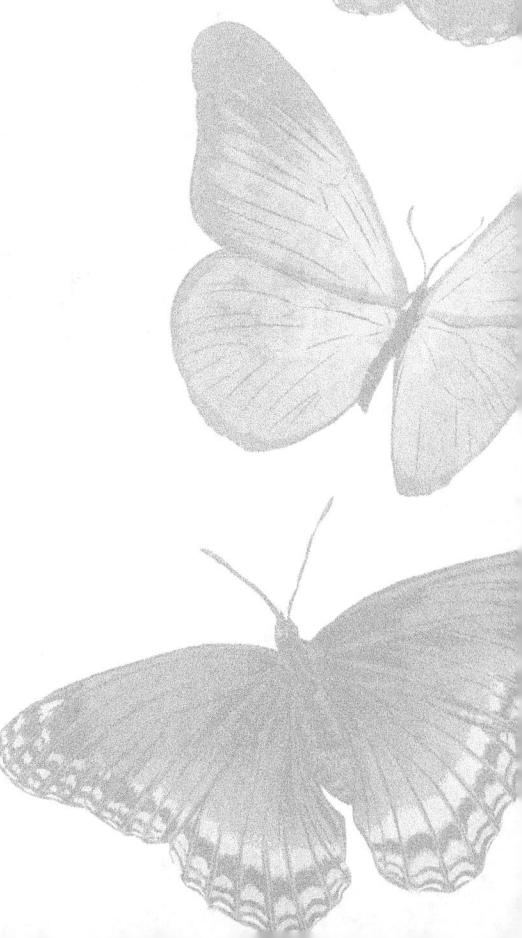

First published by Busybird Publishing 2020

Copyright © 2020 Rachel Lea

ISBN 978-1-925949-88-9

This work is copyright. Apart from any use permitted under the *Copyright Act 1968*, no part of this publication may be reproduced, stored in a retrieval system or transmitted in any form or by any means, electronic, mechanical, photocopying, recording or otherwise, without the prior written permission of Rachel Lea.

Cover Image: James Fosdike
Cover design: Busybird Publishing
Layout and typesetting: Busybird Publishing

Busybird Publishing
2/118 Para Road
Montmorency, Victoria
Australia 3094

Dedication

This book is dedicated to the following people:

To the Lupus Warriors of the world – may you always lift up, persevere and use strength, for you are not alone.

To my former students – may this book be an example of my words to you in action: anything is possible with pride and perseverance so … strive xx

For Mum, Dad and Bec – for always believing in me and lifting me up with your loving, generous hearts xxx

Contents

Foreword   i
Preface   v

Part One
Lift Up: The Diagnosis and My Support System   1
Chapter 1: Little Pinkie Finger   3
Chapter 2: Stuck in Limbo   11
Chapter 3: Diagnosis of M.E.   20
Chapter 4: What are Family and Friends For?   27
Chapter 5: Fighting Back with Scrabble and Cups of Tea   36
Chapter 6: Is It Lupus?   41
Chapter 7: Well, It Is Lupus   50
Chapter 8: So, What Is Lupus?   52

Part Two
Persevere: Adjusting to My New Normal   61
Chapter 9: So, I Have Lupus   63
Chapter 10: VCE On Steroids   69
Chapter 11: Discovering Strength in Perseverance   77
Chapter 12: Under the Radar   85
Chapter 13: Clipped Wings   98
Chapter 14: Plodding Along   107
Chapter 15: Being Lumped with More Worry   113
Chapter 16: Another Step Forward   121
Chapter 17: Achieving the Unachievable   129

Part Three
Use Strength: Living with Hope and Perspective   133
   Chapter 18: The Art of Disclosure   135
   Chapter 19: Bully for Me   149
   Chapter 20: Are You Really My Friend?   159
   Chapter 21: Here Comes the Sun   165
   Chapter 22: But Do You Know? Do You Really Know?   171
   Chapter 23: Making Lemonade out of Lemons   181
   Chapter 24: Keeping the Wolf from the Door   188

Epilogue   196
Acknowledgements   204
Author's Biography   209
Useful Resources   211
Lupus Support Services   213
Endnotes   217

Foreword

During a stressful period in my teaching career, I found myself expressing my frustrations by writing in a journal each night after a long day at school. My mind was often racing, as I tried to process and comprehend the many incidents of unkind, selfish behaviour I was witnessing within my teaching faculty and amongst the teaching staff. At the time, I was extremely unwell and struggling to make it through a day at school. I could feel myself fading, as I struggled to complete simple tasks. Watching my colleagues implement their teaching duties with ease, I was in awe of the normality of the working day for them. Seeing some of them behave with cruel, unforgiving judgement of other people exasperated me. Evidence of a safe, respectful work environment was becoming much harder to find. I was watching them waste the gifts that I believed they had been given – the gifts of good physical health and the opportunity to teach and nurture their students, by instead choosing to participate in the bullying and condemnation of their fellow colleagues. As a result, I began to feel very isolated, extremely lonely and sad.

I was constantly asking myself, 'How can I keep moving forward when I am surrounded by so much negativity? How can I find hope and purpose as a chronically ill person in a toxic work environment?' – one where people were strongly resisting the opportunity to invest more time and effort in creating greater goodwill and positive change that everyone could benefit from. How long can I endure the frustration of working like this and be able to take good care of myself and be in the best possible health? And ultimately, the question that intrigued me the most, 'How do other people, like me, who have invisible chronic illnesses, cope in stressful, challenging workplaces? How do they find their way in the world, when their pain is invisible to those around them?' These thoughts and feelings ruminated in my mind for a long time, and before I knew it, I had started to write and explore my life as a Lupus Warrior (the universal name for people who have lupus), the result of which is the production of this book.

Stress in the workplace has dominated my working life and I've always been challenged by what I would see – colleagues not being as grateful as I was, to be well, working and contributing to the world; that as a chronically ill person, I was fraught with anxiety every working day, dependent on my ability to perform my job competently and reliably. Complacency was not allowed, for my normal as a chronically ill person was not the normal for those around me. I was different. And I have found that extremely difficult to navigate.

Reflecting in this way and at this time in my life has enabled me to recognise the significance of my achievements as a Lupus Warrior and that the many stressful moments in my working life have actually been some of the greatest lessons of my life, for they have forced me to confront and take responsibility for my own growth and happiness as a person. Ultimately, I have come to learn that sharing my experiences of having lupus for the past 30 years may be of some benefit for fellow Lupus Warriors who are also struggling to find their form of normal in a stressful, often insensitive and challenging world. It is time for me to be brave, to share my story and play my role as an advocate for creating greater understanding and awareness of lupus. It is my greatest hope that this book can offer companionship and unity for my fellow Lupus Warriors in the knowledge that they are not alone, as being chronically ill in this world can sometimes generate greater challenges than the disease itself.

Conversely, I hope the experiences I share in this book can shine a light on lupus as a disease, as it demands more scientific and medical intervention than ever before. Despite the increase in prevalence of autoimmune diseases such as lupus throughout the world, it is still taking far too long for Lupus Warriors to be accurately diagnosed by the medical fraternity. As a result, irreversible organ damage, shorter life expectancy and even death are often the tragic outcomes. Minimal options for the treatment of lupus are continuing to deprive our communities of healthy, vibrant and productive members, which is equally as tragic. With greater education within our global community of what lupus is and what its symptoms are, hopefully more effective intervention and accurate diagnosis of lupus can be made so that more lives can be saved. This is my hope.

Purple is used as the colour to attract awareness to the lupus cause. Specifically, a purple butterfly is the symbol used to represent Lupus Warriors throughout the world. The extraordinary artist, James Fosdike, has kindly contributed to this book. He has created a striking illustration for the front cover, a series of stunning purple butterflies circling my face, in recognition of lupus and Lupus Warriors around the world. So, whenever you see a purple butterfly, please think of the millions of Lupus Warriors persevering each day. Please remember us, support us and help to lift us up, so that we can truly fly.

Rachel Lea,
Lupus Warrior

Preface

As a child growing up, I could be described as many things. Creative, academic, physically active, thoughtful, mature for my age; but the words that would be used to describe me the most would be quiet and shy. I was capable of socialising with my friends, but I was also very happy to spend time in my own company.

I was an extremely creative child and would spend hours painting and sketching. I was very inspired by my grandpa, Pa, who was an outstanding painter. He painted beautiful pictures of Australian homesteads and native fauna including gum trees and flowers. Iconic Australian wildlife, such as koalas and kookaburras, were also his favourites to paint. I wanted to draw and paint just like him. I would paint on canvas or in my huge A3 sketchbook. I would often use Pa's paintings as images that I would then try and emulate myself. Pa taught me how to use charcoal to sketch with and how to use the myriad of paintbrushes for just the right effect. Trees and butterflies were my favourite objects to draw. I would just lose myself in this creative space and could be found painting or sketching whenever time permitted. I would sit outside under the pergola in our backyard and enjoy the stillness that drawing brings. Tapestry and anything crafty with glue were also my hobbies during childhood. Like painting, I loved having a blank slate with which to begin creating a picture. The concentration of the fine needle work would centre me and also keep me busy.

If I wasn't painting, doing needle work or sticking something together with craft glue, I could be found reading. A self-confessed bookworm, I could quite happily disappear into a book for hours. I always looked forward to our family trips to the local library, where I would return home with the maximum number of books that I was able to borrow each month. I so enjoyed escaping into one story after another, and the sense of achievement in finishing each book gave me a feeling of fulfilment, of time well spent.

Whilst these activities were quite sedentary, I was also very physically active as a child. I loved getting out into our garden and helping my Dad with the weeding and the pruning. I enjoyed the feeling and sensation of getting my hands in the dirt, the sun shining down on me and the satisfaction of turning an overgrown, weed-riddled patch of garden into a restored vision of calm and order. There was one particular spot in the garden that I saw as a challenge and that was weeding the thick ivy creeper that was sprawled across most of our back fence. Weeds would shoot up thick, fast and tall throughout the ivy, and I would see this as my job to get rid of them all so that the gorgeous ivy leaves could be seen in all of their glory. I could be found outside weeding in our backyard for hours – more specifically, until the job was done. Helping in the garden was never a chore for pocket money. I just wanted to help and to be in nature.

In my opinion, I was also a self-awarded bat tennis champion, endurance bike rider and super tree climber! Hayaki, which was a very physical game of hide-and-seek created by the kids in our court, neighbourhood cricket and kicking the footy were also in the mix. I felt so energised and free, mucking around doing these things with my older brother Ross, younger sister Rebecca and other kids in our quiet, suburban court until dark, when it was always time to come inside. When each morning came, I couldn't wait to start the day. I would be up at 6 am and eager to get to school. So eager that I would arrive at school an hour early so that I could help the teachers, particularly in the library, searching for lost books or processing new ones. My dream was to become a teacher. I adored everything about my teachers and had a strong sense that I could one day be one too. At this young and precious age, I always had a sense of purpose and wanting to help others. I also just loved doing things that made me happy, and looking back now, I feel much comfort that I lived my childhood days well. Without realising it, I was true to myself even then. Just being me and getting the most out of each day.

I was also a very grateful child. I recognised that any gift I received was a special item to always be treasured. Whilst I would happily use my charcoal and paints to sketch and paint with, I would lovingly admire but rarely use my Derwent pencils – rich, vibrant colours perfectly sharpened and lined up in a neat row inside their specially designed tin. They would be displayed carefully on my bedroom desk. I saw these pencils as an expensive gift – never to be wasted on rough drawings. If I were to use them, it was sporadically and only for very special occasions. I was the same with other gifts. Gorgeous soaps, bath bombs and shower gels were more like ornaments, as I rarely used them. Always beautifully wrapped and shining in their freshness, I enjoyed creating pretty displays for them on my dresser. They too were to be savoured and never to be wasted. Bottles of perfumes that I also received as gifts were carefully organised and placed on my dresser as well – their fragrances rarely released for they too were to be used sparingly, if at all, and again only for special occasions.

* * *

As I entered my teenage years, more specifically around the age of fourteen, the freedom of reading a much-loved book, riding my bike or painting a picture whenever I wished, became distant memories of another life lived. Over time, I didn't have the physical strength to hold a book, let alone the concentration needed to read or understand it. Riding my bike became an impossible task. I had little to no energy or strength in my muscles to will my body forward with the physical movement needed to keep those wheels turning. I could no longer be in the direct rays of the sun. I would develop fevers, instant fatigue, severe headaches and red, blotchy rashes on my face, arms and legs if I stood outside in the direct sunlight or in the line of ultraviolet (UV) rays for longer than five-to-ten minutes. This meant that I was unable to garden during the day in the beautiful sunlight.

Over time, I no longer felt like painting or sketching. I wasn't interested. If I did feel the inclination to draw, I found it extremely difficult to hold the brush – my hands swollen in joint pain and chilblains. I would stare long and hard at what I wanted to sketch but struggled to find the connection between my hand and my mind that would allow me to create that image. That natural fine motor movement was slow and unsteady. The creative spark – gone.

LUPUS = *Lift Up, Persevere, Use Strength*

I was no longer bursting out of bed at 6 am anymore. Getting up early became impossible, as excessive fatigue left my body feeling such a deep heaviness that much effort was needed as I struggled to get up and out of bed. What was happening to me? Why was I experiencing such pain and fatigue? Why had I become so different, so fragile and so scared? A mysterious disease that not many people had heard of, systemic lupus erythematosus, had entered my body. The freedom of my world changed infinitely.

Disease is such a scary word. It even sounds contagious – inescapable. Like it's reaching out, trying to grab you. Whether it's heard through the spoken word or seen in writing, it lingers and permeates. Most of all, it instils fear. To be told as a young person that you have a disease was simply terrifying. So many diseases receive elaborate, headlining attention through either larger prevalence or savvy, memorable marketing campaigns; those are the diseases that most people can recognise and understand – cancer, multiple sclerosis, heart disease, to name a few. The frightening, looming diseases that take lives. Their cures are promoted and celebrated as the most important; needed more desperately to stop these diseases in their tracks.

Then there is the group of diseases that attract little, if any, attention. The ones that don't have the numbers. The minority. These diseases are often difficult to pronounce and difficult to remember. They make little impact and generate little fuss, particularly if they don't always cause high numbers of death. These diseases are likely to be chronic, incurable diseases yet seemingly invisible to the naked eye. Systemic lupus erythematosus is one of these diseases. To remember how to say it is a triumph, to spell it, an achievement, and to overcome it, a miracle, for there is currently no cure for this disease that I, and millions of others around the world, suffer from. It belongs to the many forgotten or unheard of invisible chronic illnesses of which so many people aren't aware.

When you read the many stories of the suffering of others, it's hard to view your own struggles objectively. Well, at least I do. The likely response is comparing your own pain and suffering to the pain and suffering experienced by others. This can stop you from recognising the true strength and courage you have demonstrated to those around you but not fully recognised within yourself. Everyone else's journey in overcoming adversity can seem more important, more significant, than your own story. How can battling something like a chronic illness even compare to fighting cancer or overcoming life-changing disability through injury?

Preface

How can my experience as a lupus sufferer generate any interest when my biggest achievement is simply living through what would appear to be a regular day; navigating a world where many people don't know how lucky they are to live a so-called 'normal' life.

During the thirty years I have suffered from this disease, I've realised that I am being extremely unfair to myself by dismissing my struggle as nothing extraordinary. I have finally learnt that my story does matter, as do the stories of millions of lupus sufferers throughout the world. More and more of our voices are becoming heard as lupus awareness and education increase by the day. We are known as Lupus Warriors, for we have much courage and are determined that the quality of our lives to live well will always have great purpose and meaning, despite suffering from lupus.

When I think of how lupus has changed me and my approach to life, it has been more of a cumulative shift in how I have evolved. Ageing and maturity have been significant contributing factors in how I respond to either new or existing lupus challenges. I like to think that I have developed greater empathy and more awareness of the suffering and struggles of others. I listen with more attentiveness and try not to be judgemental. I try to be more thoughtful and caring in all that I do. I find that I am always reflecting on my life and how well I am living it.

I'm often asking myself questions, such as am I happy with the choices and decisions I am making? Am I being true to myself in all that I do? Am I doing everything I can do to be as well as I can be? Am I being kinder to myself, as opposed to being too hard on myself, if I haven't completed an important task? Why? For I must have purpose and fulfilment in everything I do. Every day must count. Sweating the small stuff is simply not allowed because if I do and get caught up in trivial, petty problems then I will be wasting the life lessons being ill is trying to teach me. And to me, that would be shameful.

Compared with my childhood, when anything special I received was treasured and rarely used, in my life today, I don't leave those pencils lined up, neat, tidy and untouched anymore. I use every single one them. I don't let those soaps sit unused in pretty displays. When I receive them, I immediately rip them open from their packaging and lather them up with gratitude. I drop those bath bombs into warm, soothing water and make sure that I feel every bubble, every tingle and all of the fizz. And I dust off those perfume bottles, pop their lids and deeply inhale their beautiful aromas. I use every drop of that perfume until I'm ready for the next bottle.

Part One

Lift Up

The Diagnosis and My Support System

Chapter One

Little Pinkie Finger

My little pinkie finger on my left hand started it. Cheeky finger! To be exact, a strange, red and itchy lump on my left pinkie finger. It was a pesky little thing. I would scratch it so much that I just wanted to rip it off my hand. It was May 1989 and I was in Year 8 at secondary school. I was thirteen years old. After a couple of months of itching and scratching, I eventually mentioned it to my parents. On inspection, they said that it was a chilblain. I had never heard of chilblains. So off we went to the chemist to get some chilblain tablets that were meant to relieve me of this little annoyance. After a couple of months of taking these tablets, more chilblains began appearing on my hands. I was taking about nine chilblain tablets a day, which would leave me experiencing nasty hot flushes and a face full of red blotches.

The temperature of my hands also began to change. Despite being inflamed with these chilblains, my hands became extremely cold to touch. They started to change colour, mostly red and purple. Completing my schoolwork was a challenge. It was very painful to hold a pen. My right thumb was very swollen, particularly at the base where the movement of holding a pen presses on the bone. Actually, it was excruciating. Thankfully, the chemist had long rolls of a product called tubey foam. It was literally a thin roll of pink foam with a gauze lining on the inside of the roll. I would cut this foam into suitable lengths for my thumb and fingers. I would then place them on my thumb and first two fingers to cushion my joints and chilblains from rubbing directly onto the pen. This helped me to hold a pen, but it was still painful and challenging to create a writing style that flowed. It took me much longer to complete my work. I persevered and ignored the stares and jibes from classmates and just got on with it as best I could. In all honesty, I felt grateful that we had found a way so that I was able to write.

* * *

Prior to the September school holidays in 1989 and still battling cold hands and chilblains, I started to feel different. Not myself at all. I remember having quite a lot of homework and I couldn't handle any of it. Very out of character for a studious girl such as myself. I was walking around jabbering words such as, 'I'm going to crack, I'm going to crack'. Eventually, I did. I remember screaming, yelling and crying so hard that I couldn't stop. After a day of continual crying, Mum called for our family GP (general practitioner) to visit me at home. I needed to be sedated. Mum put me to bed and told me that I wouldn't be returning to school until after the holidays. My mood improved over the holidays as I rested and took it easy.

Upon returning to school, I remember not feeling right. I felt tired and weak. I went to school anyway and, would you believe, on the first day back, it was my turn to do yard duty for the whole day! I told the teacher that I wasn't feeling well and asked if I could be relieved from completing the yard duty. The answer was no and I was made to wander around the entire school yard, holding a huge rubbish bin and filling it up with disgusting rubbish. I was such an obedient student. I simply accepted that I wasn't allowed to sit this out and did what I was told, regardless of how I was feeling. I don't know how I managed to finish the yard duty, but I did – at a cost. A huge cost. I felt awful. I was absolutely exhausted. My entire body felt heavy, sore and painful. I could barely stand up or walk. I practically crawled home from school and collapsed onto the lounge room floor when I finally made the long journey home. Mum picked me up and put me to bed. She and Dad were distraught. They were so angry with the teacher at school for making me pick up rubbish when I had said that I was unwell.

I continued to feel this way the following day. I had never felt this sick before. Extremely concerned, my parents booked me in to see a local paediatrician. I had to wait a couple of months for my appointment with him. In the meantime, I was still quite fatigued, very pale and experiencing achy joints and muscles. I was sleeping a lot during the day and had lost a lot of weight. I had little strength and needed the aid of a walking stick to move around the house. Subsequently, I was absent from school for the remainder of the year.

When it finally came time to see the paediatrician, I had mixed feelings about his appraisal of my symptoms. The consult began with the paediatrician, an old, tall and foreboding man, performing an extremely thorough but invasive physical examination of me. I remember the consulting room being very small, with a window so high up that it could not be gazed out of, and it was so dark and cold. I was all alone with this strange man. Lying on the examination bed in my bra and undies was extremely confronting for me. I had never been to the hospital or been majorly ill in my life, so to have a doctor physically examine my body in this way was new and quite scary. I had only just turned fourteen. Such a self-conscious and delicate age. This physical examination felt like it would never end. It felt like I was being physically dissected. My weight and height were recorded and analysed. Even my menstruation cycle was discussed.

Once the physical examination was finished, I was then asked to put my clothes back on and to sit down on the chair opposite the doctor at his desk. The consultation then shifted gears. It went from being a physical examination to a counselling session with the paediatrician. He began to analyse the state of my mental health. I was bombarded with a range of very personal questions. I was asked to share my thoughts on family members, friends, school and myself. He spent a lot of time questioning me about my eating habits, and I felt as though he was implying that I had an eating disorder. I found this extremely hard. The physical examination was intrusive enough and, in many ways, traumatic. I had no time to digest how I felt about experiencing this. I was then expected to sit in front of the doctor immediately after this physical examination and share my inner-most thoughts with him after he had practically seen me naked and touched most of my body; it was simply too much. I found myself being very vague and evasive with my answers. I did not want to participate in this process at all. Somehow, I answered his questions the best way I could and got through it. The doctor then called my parents into the room and, relieved that this part of the consultation was over, I then sat outside and waited for his verdict.

As the paediatrician was giving my parents his appraisal of my symptoms, he scrutinised their parenting skills with a barrage of questions about my weight loss. The paediatrician felt very strongly that I was suffering from an eating disorder that both my parents were unaware. My parents felt that they were on trial. The paediatrician was especially hard on Mum. She felt that he was implying that she was not an observant, caring mother because, if she was, she would be able to recognise that I was hiding an eating disorder, whether it be anorexia or bulimia. Mum was outraged. She was my primary carer and was with me all day, every day. Mum was preparing my meals, bathing me, helping me in and out of bed when my fatigue was that extreme, and she even needed to feed me herself when I lacked strength to feed myself. She would be the first person to notice if I was not eating much, skipping meals or worse, running to the toilet to throw up any food I'd eaten.

For the paediatrician to misjudge my parents as ignorant or neglectful was uncalled for. Anger quickly rose in Mum, and she recalls wanting to punch him on the nose! Without hesitation, Mum went into mother bear mode and challenged the doctor in a very heated verbal exchange to defend our family. Dad was more pensive in digesting the paediatrician's comments. I couldn't ask for more loving, caring parents, and to know that they were put under the microscope that way makes me sad – even to this day.

As frustrating as it was for my parents, they could recognise the sensitive nature of this issue. If the paediatrician genuinely suspected that I had an eating disorder, it was his duty of care as a physician to delve further into the issue. He had an obligation to report my parents to the relevant child welfare authorities if he strongly suspected that my parents were negligent in the care of their daughter. Whilst Mum and Dad strongly rejected the notion that I was suffering from a secret eating disorder, they had to concede and respect that this was how the paediatrician was assessing my health at this time. Personally, I felt angry. My inexplicable symptoms of physical pain were being overlooked in favour of the examination of my eating behaviours. Surely, the combination of physical pain, fatigue and weight loss, implied that something more sinister was happening.

In regard to the physical symptoms of extreme fatigue, joint and muscle pain I was experiencing at the time, and considering the fact that I was a quiet but dedicated and studious student, the paediatrician diagnosed me with burnout and stress from working too hard at school. I remember feeling very frustrated at hearing this. I felt judged. Yes, I worked hard at school. It always mattered to me that I did my best in all of my subjects, even the ones I didn't like or wasn't that good at. But I was not a perfectionist or someone with unrealistic expectations of what I could achieve. I had a balanced life outside of school. How I could be burnt out at the age of fourteen truly baffled me. Yes, I was stressed out. I felt stressed out because I felt sick and I was worried about myself – about what was causing me to feel this way. Surely, this was a normal, completely understandable reaction to what was happening to me. Inexplicably, I was losing weight, had extremely cold yet swollen hands and constant chilblains, was extremely tired and had achy joints and muscles. I was no doctor, but I couldn't help but feel something was seriously wrong with me based on these physical symptoms alone. How on earth could stress and burnout cause these symptoms? How could I be losing all of this weight, even though I was eating normally? Admittedly, the paediatrician did concede that he did not know what was causing my cold hands and chilblains, and he referred me to see a professor of paediatric rheumatology at the Royal Children's Hospital in Melbourne. It would be another long wait in this journey of finding answers to my health worries.

With more thought and discussion after this consultation, my parents agreed that they would allow me to continue seeing the paediatrician, even though my parents strongly disagreed with him that a suspected eating disorder was the cause of my weight loss. The pathology tests I had been routinely completing all continued to indicate that I was a healthy young woman. The paediatrician was also a highly regarded physician and qualified teenage psychiatrist. My parents felt that maybe the cause of my physical aches and pains were symptoms of stress and burnout, given that my test results indicated that I was in good health. They felt that the paediatrician may be able to address any underlying mental health issues I may be suffering from in an attempt to explain the cause of my symptoms and to ultimately help in improving my overall health. So, the plan was this: I would see the paediatrician regularly so that he would take care of my mental state, and in the meantime, I would wait to see the professor in the hopes that he could find the cause of my cold hands and chilblains.

The regular counselling sessions with the paediatrician began. The thought of me being alone in a room with this doctor terrified me, and I absolutely hated every minute of these sessions. However, I put up a good front and cooperated with this agonising process. The doctor continued to focus on my mental state and asked me very personal questions. I had great difficulty sharing my feelings in this space. I was expected to discuss my feelings about family, friends and school and in particular how I felt about myself. I could sense that he was looking for possible evidence of low self-esteem and distorted body image issues with his constant questions focusing on my eating habits. He would frequently discuss my weight. He informed me that I was too thin for my height and that I needed to put on another 5 kilograms. This was distressing for me as I was eating regularly, not missing meals and nor did I have any issues with my appearance. I didn't want to share any of my real feelings, so I would tell the odd white lie here and there to get through it. Anything to hurry these sessions along so that I could get out of that cold, dark and invasive room.

I could feel my resentment at being probed in this way escalating into anger as I just felt so alone and so frustrated that I was being psychoanalysed. This paediatrician was not interested in actively seeking the answers to my physical symptoms of lethargy and joint and muscle pain. He was not interested in my cold, chilblain-riddled hands at all. My account of this pain and suffering was being dismissed and not deemed as legitimate or as genuine. Resolving the true cause of my physical suffering was not a priority. I felt completely disempowered and at the mercy of grown-ups – the paediatrician, my GP and even my parents.

***

Towards the end of 1989, my appointment with the professor of paediatric rheumatology at the Royal Children's Hospital arrived. Upon meeting the professor, I recall him being a warm, friendly man. He was a much, much older man than the paediatrician and was clearly ready for retirement, but he was very intrigued with my symptoms and my case in general. Clinically, all of my blood tests continued to indicate that I was normal. No sign of disease. Completely healthy. I found this very frustrating. My parents were just as frustrated and extremely worried. I was not wishing myself to be ill or diseased. I just wanted a name, something tangible to make sense of my symptoms. To find a way to ease my pain with treatment and, if possible, a cure. Something to confirm that I was not making up these symptoms. My pain was very real and not self-inflicted.

The professor was at a loss to describe the cause of my cold hands and chilblains. I had long stopped taking the chilblain tablets due to side effects of hot flushes. They were not successful in treating or reducing the number of chilblains anyway. The professor thought that my symptoms of fatigue and joint and muscle pain were the result of either a virus or physical exhaustion. He referred me to a rheumatologist in the hope that he was able to determine the cause of my cold hands and chilblains. He was extremely sorry that he was unable to give us more definitive answers. He could see how worried we all were. I remember feeling comforted by the fact that this professor really cared. My suffering was being acknowledged.

Visiting the rheumatologist continued to be another frustrating experience in the quest to find answers. He was a tall, thin and very conservative middle-aged man, and the one memory that Dad has of this doctor was his appearance; always wearing crisply starched and non-creased shirts. He conveyed a seriousness that said, 'Don't waste my time.' The rheumatologist was a minimalist in his appraisal of my symptoms. Again, my pathology tests continued to be normal, and he concluded that I simply had a severe case of chilblains. He struggled to describe the cause of my extremely cold hands and concocted the term 'Acute Vascular Instability Syndrome' to help give these symptoms a name and some meaning. He instructed me to wear gloves to keep my hands warm at all times. He told me that I wasn't as sick as I thought I was and that I would get better soon and didn't need to see him again.

Not as sick as I thought I was. Again, the symptoms of fatigue, muscular aches, joint pains and weight loss I was experiencing were dismissed as signs of anything serious. I continued to feel extremely confused and frustrated as to why these symptoms were not being examined more urgently. It felt strange to have this doctor invent a name to justify my pain. I remember feeling very insignificant and that finding a cause and, if possible, a cure to my suffering was not being seen as an important challenge to solve by the medical community supposedly charged to take care of me.

The lack of urgency to help make me feel better by this doctor contributed to an already isolating time for me. The loneliness I was experiencing in this situation was much like my physical pain; completely debilitating. I did not know anyone suffering in the way I was. I had no one to talk to and share my pain with. This was a time well before internet forums and blogs were accessible. No Facebook to reach out to others who were suffering like me. However, as my symptoms didn't have a real name, there was no starting place to reach out from or to seek emotional support from anyway. I felt truly helpless, and I know my parents did too. My friends from school didn't visit me at home. There were maybe the odd phone calls but generally school life for my peers continued to roll on without me. With the love and encouragement from my parents, brother and sister, I simply did my best to keep resting and get through each day the best I could with the hope that somehow my health would improve.

Chapter Two

Stuck in Limbo

Amazingly, my degree of fatigue, achiness and lack of energy had improved to a point where I was able to return to school full-time in 1990. I was in Year 9, turning fifteen years old. However, I still battled cold, painful hands and chilblains. I continued to find completing schoolwork extremely difficult. I still needed my tubey foam on my writing fingers to cushion the swelling and I wore fingerless gloves to improve the temperature of my hands because they were still so cold and red and purple in colour. Then one day, pain spread into my hands. An aching that was constant. Heavy. The joints around my knuckles had become more intensely swollen and red. On one occasion, I remember asking, 'Mum, can you please, please cut off my hands?' They were hurting so much. My poor Mum. All she could do was give me a cuddle and the reassurance that, hopefully, the doctors could relieve my pain somehow. I had this overwhelming feeling of wanting to be rid of my hands – for someone to take them away, so that I could feel lighter and pain-free.

Regular sessions with the paediatrician continued, and as these sessions progressed, my parents became more frustrated that my key physical symptoms were not being acknowledged by the doctor, as the focus on my mental health intensified with each appointment. After much discussion, thankfully, they agreed that I no longer had to continue seeing the paediatrician. Wow, was I relieved! They could see how distressed I was before and after these sessions. This was a form of extra, undue stress for me, and my parents felt that seeing the paediatrician was not good for my health, let alone helping to provide the myriad of answers as to why I was feeling so sick.

As the pain in my hands spread and even more chilblains appeared, the deterioration of these symptoms was of much concern for my parents. The stabbing and aching pains that had developed were chronic and unrelenting. I couldn't straighten my hands or fingers at all, and I could barely hold a pen, let alone write with it. Participating in written tasks at school was excruciating. I found grasping and holding onto objects very hard, and I was constantly dropping and smashing things as a result. Whilst the physical aches and fatigue I had experienced previously appeared to have eased, I was still tired after a day at school. I was still very pale and thin.

My parents decided to arrange for me to see the rheumatologist again to seek his opinion on these changes. Upon my return visit, he commented that my hands looked 'quite nasty'. Whilst I explained the stabbing and aching pain I was experiencing, he said that although it sounded like arthritis, it wasn't, because my bone tissues did not appear to be damaged. From his physical examination of my hands, he said that the blood tissues around my bones were swollen, which was causing all of the pain. He said that my blood wasn't flowing correctly into my hands and that was why my hands were as cold as ice all of the time. The chilblains had developed because of the chronic coldness in my hands. I was given no definitive diagnosis, aside from the concocted name of 'Acute Vascular Instability Syndrome'. My symptoms still had no proper name. To help ease the pain, the rheumatologist prescribed an anti-inflammatory medication and recommended that I continue seeing him on a regular basis to monitor these symptoms.

And so that is what we did. I made routine visits to the rheumatologist throughout 1990. He was quite a moody doctor. Sometimes he was seemingly caring and sympathetic to my plight, at other times, he was very abrupt and dismissive. The anti-inflammatory medication was mildly helpful, only relieving some of the pain. As the year progressed, my hands continued to be super cold and full of chilblains. I was still feeling tired after school, but on the rare occasion, I was able to participate in regular physical activity such as swimming and aerobics. It felt wonderful to be active when I was well enough, and it boosted my spirits considerably.

One of my favourite teachers at school, my Food Technology teacher, Karen Bryce, knew that Mum didn't drive. In wanting to support me during this challenging time, she kindly offered to drive me home whenever I was feeling unwell during the school day. Karen gave me a copy of her teaching timetable and highlighted the spaces that were her non-teaching periods. If I was unwell during those periods, she was able to drive me home. I did call on her to drive me home a couple of times when I couldn't make it through the school day. Mum and Dad were so grateful for her generosity and compassion, as was I. My parents, all these years later, still speak of how much they appreciate her support. Karen and I became good friends and remain so to this day.

* * *

During one of my visits to the rheumatologist, Mum enquired as to whether he had any idea of what I was actually suffering from. Could he give us a clue as to any possibilities for the cause of my symptoms? The rheumatologist was quite affronted by this question and replied that he couldn't name any possible diseases that could be the cause because he needed clinical proof of disease – specifically pathology results. As my pathology results had continued to report that everything was normal, he could not say, even if he had an idea, what he thought it could be. He made the comment, quite emphatically, that if he disclosed what he suspected was the cause of my symptoms, and he was in fact wrong, we could sue him. It was a very tense conversation and a moment of desperation on Mum's part as she simply wanted to have an idea of what was wrong with me. She was pleading with the rheumatologist for not only a more definitive answer but for greater compassion for the situation she and my father were experiencing. My parents were quite offended too as legal proceedings would not be a course of action they would take if an incorrect diagnosis was made. They just wanted possible answers. They wanted to know what was ailing their once happy, vibrant and healthy girl.

My parents and I were feeling quite tired of not having even an inkling of what was wrong and the rheumatologist's unwillingness to share his medical opinion felt like another roadblock to finding answers. It was cruel as we all felt that when we left his office that day, the rheumatologist had a very strong idea of what was wrong with me, but without the clinical evidence to back him up, he was not prepared to share his opinion. You could sense his frustration as evidenced in his outburst. Well, he wasn't the only one who was frustrated. But, being the gentle, amiable people that we were (and still are), my parents and I accepted the difficulties of the rheumatologist's position and understood the ramifications of sharing a diagnosis that may not be accurate.

* * *

Whilst continuing to complete pathology tests and seeing the rheumatologist in 1990, another stressful issue arose during this time. Life at school was becoming very challenging. One of the subjects I was to complete was called Information Technology, also known as computer class. With my swollen, red and rigidly painful hands, I was absolutely dreading this class. I could barely write, let alone type. One of the major skills to achieve in completing this class was to be competent in touch-type and type a certain number of words per minute. I knew from the get-go that I was not going to be a high-flyer in this class. To make matters worse, our teacher was one of the most disliked teachers at our school. An overweight, long-bearded, grumpy and rude man who delighted in tormenting his students with his threatening, belittling manner. He was an absolute bully and we, as his students, despised him. While disciplining the class, one of his favourite lines was, 'My attitude towards you is zero.' He would enjoy slowly pacing up and down the computer aisles of our classroom, rattling the large set of keys he had dangling from his low-riding jean belt, which was struggling to hold up his bulging belly, hovering over us as we desperately tried to type our fastest.

In preparation for my first class in this subject, my parents had written a letter for this teacher, outlining the condition of my hands in conjunction with a medical certificate from my rheumatologist. They were concerned about my ability to fully participate in this class and were seeking support from this teacher in acknowledging that I had legitimate reasons for not being able to type well but that I would do my best. My parents were requesting that my medical condition be taken into consideration when it came time to formally assess me in this subject. Upon receipt of these letters from me at the beginning of this class, he stood there and read them silently in front of me. When he finished reading, he grunted, put the letters aside and walked off. Not the response a student deserving of special consideration needed.

As a shy, gentle girl with a medical condition, I was loath to seek his help after this reaction. When these classes began, I would sit there quietly and anxiously. I couldn't keep up. I was afraid to seek his help – not that he would provide it willingly anyway. He could see that I was struggling and would not offer to assist me. Worst of all, he would mock me about not being able to keep up with the rest of the class. All of my classmates raced through the typing exercises with much speed and confidence. When we completed the test that scored how many words we could type per minute, mine was a dismal score of two words per minute. *Two!* By the end of the semester, I had progressed to nine words per minute. Progress, nonetheless! I found it really, really hard to keep my fingers spread out on the keyboard and aligned in the correct way, which would enable me to speed type. I would come home from school a bit depressed about my struggles with typing, but I knew it wasn't my fault. I just didn't want to attract any extra attention from my classmates for not being able to complete something as basic as typing skills that was seemingly so easy for them. I battled on, did my best during class to complete the set tasks, but I felt despondent and disengaged.

When it came time for the semester reports to come out, I wondered what mine would say for Information Technology. I remember not being too worried as even though this teacher was a bully, I had provided him with the appropriate medical information to explain why I was likely to underperform in this class. I was confident that I would not be penalised for my inability to type quickly. To my horror, and my parents' horror, this teacher had awarded me an 'NA', or Non-Assessed, for the semester. Back then, an NA was deemed as a fail. However, today it means that a student has not been assessed according to set standards due to absences or special consideration, such as illness. His comments on the report were as follows:

> *'Rachel has been unable to complete any of the set work or goals, even on a basic level, in this subject this semester. The Touch-Typing Tutorial is still incomplete. I find it very difficult to assess Rachel because of this. Therefore, I have been forced to give her a Non-Assessed for this semester. In class she is quiet and cooperative.'*

He was *forced* to give me this grade. Not one of these comments in the report acknowledged my medical condition. The teacher had been given not only a written account from my parents but also a medical certificate – not from a GP but from a specialist. The comments implied that I was a lazy student who had shown no effort in trying to participate in this class. For this teacher to completely disregard prior notification of my medical condition was astounding. It felt like an act of discrimination. To state that I had not completed any set work or goals was an absolute lie; I had not refused any work and had tried my hardest to complete all set goals. My parents were shocked and angry that I had been treated this way. Their efforts to be proactive in seeking support for their daughter were completely dismissed.

Initially, my parents fought very hard to organise a time to meet with the school principal to discuss this matter. Unfortunately, they were repeatedly given the run-around. Dad would seek permission to leave work (he worked as a project manager at Melbourne Airport) so that he could attend an organised meeting with the principal, only to arrive home to pick up Mum and be called on the phone at the last minute, informed that the meeting was cancelled. This happened a few times. My poor Dad had been taking so much time off work to drive me to all of my medical appointments, so to be disrespected like this was extremely frustrating and stressful for him. My parents decided to take this issue a step further by seeking support from our local Department of Education Region. They were very sympathetic to our plight and awarded a liaison officer to act on behalf of my parents in communications with the principal.

After much delay, the liaison officer helped my parents to finally have a meeting with the school principal to discuss the report. It was my parents' wish for the principal to be supportive of me and of my right to have this report rewritten to acknowledge my limitations but also to acknowledge my efforts in completing the set work. They were also seeking their right to have me, as their child, taken out of this teacher's class. It was this request that had the principal fuming. He was a very stubborn and easily agitated man, bordering on retirement. He was extremely offended that my parents were demanding that I be taken out of this teacher's class. He insisted that I must attend his class as per Department of Education guidelines at that time. Eventually, the principal conceded that the written report could have been worded differently.

After a somewhat heated discussion, it was agreed that another meeting with my parents, the principal and the teacher involved would be arranged as soon as possible to resolve these issues. The principal also reassured my parents that he would seek me out at school to speak with me personally about these issues. Unfortunately, it was expected at this time that I was to continue attending this teacher's class.

My parents waited and waited for another meeting to be arranged but heard nothing from the principal. Neither did the principal organise a time to speak with me personally about these issues. Dad finally rang the principal, only to be told that he would ring Dad back with a time and date for the proposed meeting. Five weeks had passed and still nothing. So, my parents took their fight to the highest power – the State Education Minister for Victoria. They wrote a long, compelling letter regarding these issues to the Minister and in reply received notification from the Minister's secretary that he was investigating the matter.

My parents were extremely worried about my health and how the delay by the principal in resolving these issues was affecting me. I had been advised by my rheumatologist to reduce stress as much as possible, and the longer this issue went unresolved, the more stressful it became. At this time, I was starting the second semester of school. I was being mistreated by the same Information Technology teacher in his class whilst these discussions with the principal were taking place. On one occasion, I was standing in a line of three students, waiting to be handed some computer disks by the teacher. Then another line, a longer one, also formed in the classroom full of students also waiting for these disks. The teacher decided to serve every single student in this longer line before ours. He then served the two students ahead of me. He stopped when it came to my turn and served a couple of students who had formed another line. Finally, when there were no more students lined up, he served me. He had made a very pointed effort of serving every single student ahead of me.

On another occasion I was in line waiting to hand in an assignment to this teacher. As soon as I reached the front of the line, he turned around and went to make himself a cup of coffee in a room adjacent to our classroom, firmly shutting the door. I waited, then knocked on the door twice. No answer. He eventually came out, and whilst I was still standing there patiently waiting, he snatched the assignment from me. These tense and awkward exchanges made me feel extremely uncomfortable, vulnerable and full of despair.

In December of that year, my parents finally received a letter from the liaison officer from the local Department of Education Region representing my parents. He informed my parents that he had met with the principal and teacher concerned on behalf of the Minister for Education. He had successfully arranged for my Semester One Information Technology report to be rewritten to include satisfactory comments and acknowledgement of work completed and also for myself and my siblings not to be placed into any of this teacher's classes whilst we were students at this school. Progress at last! My parents and I felt relief that the principal was finally being cooperative. The liaison officer had also arranged a final meeting between my parents, the principal and the teacher, where my parents were to personally receive the rewritten report.

Whilst it appeared that we were making progress, my parents were very apprehensive about attending this meeting with the principal and the teacher as they were yet to receive, in writing, any communication from the Minister for Education to support the arrangements made by the liaison officer acting on his behalf. Unfortunately, they had good cause to be apprehensive as when the meeting finally arrived, all throughout the meeting, the teacher sat cowardly in the corner and only spoke when he was spoken to. The principal reprimanded my parents for taking this matter to the Minister for Education. On top of that, the rewritten report that he promised was apparently 'misplaced and sitting somewhere' on the principal's messy desk. During this meeting, there was no effort made by the principal to locate the rewritten report on his desk. However, the teacher did offer to reprint the report. The principal insisted that my parents would receive it as soon as possible in the mail.

Throughout this whole experience, my parents were extremely shocked and disappointed by how I was treated by this teacher and the principal. It was very distressing to experience such ignorance and a lack of compassion for our plight. We were not asking for much. All we wished for was that I was treated fairly as a student in this class, for some slight modifications and concessions to be made to my assessment as I aimed to give my best effort possible. My parents did not need this extra stress and neither did I, particularly at a time when there were still no definitive answers to explain my ill health. My parents were exhausted by how long they had to fight for this wrong to be righted. To leave the meeting that day without holding that report in their hands was beyond frustrating.

At the beginning of the school year in 1991, I had unfortunately been placed into this teacher's class again, even though it had been agreed that neither myself nor my siblings were to be placed in his classes ever again. Weary and frustrated by this seemingly never-ending issue, but not without resolve, my parents put pen to paper and continued fighting for their right to have the Minister for Education's decisions upheld and implemented. And what about the rewritten report from the year before? We have never seen it. Unfortunately, we had to let the fight for justice in these matters go, for the new year ahead, 1991, brought more challenges that became a higher priority for my parents and me to battle with. The biggest we had ever faced.

Chapter Three

Diagnosis of M.E.

I remember sitting in class and just gazing long and dreamily out of the window. The teacher's voice just drifted into the background. It was the beginning of the new school year, Year 10 English class, 1991, and I had no interest at all in the new novel we were about to study. I would long for the school bell to ring after each class, as this meant one step closer to home time. I couldn't concentrate in any of my classes, was easily distracted and even started talking and messing about with other students. This was not how the studious, conscientious Miss Rachel Lea behaved at all. When I did get home from school, I would do anything but my homework. I was simply not interested and clearly not myself. On top of these feelings, I was tired. A day at school made me really tired.

When I did get around to starting my homework, I would struggle to make sense of what I was writing. Everything felt jumbled up. I couldn't seem to spell simple words and I'd find it difficult to construct sentences and answer questions. No wonder I didn't want to do my homework. I also didn't feel happy within myself. I would appear happy and carefree on the surface, but inside, I'd become depressed too easily over small, silly things. I concluded that I was feeling this way due to back-to-school nerves, but somewhere in the back of my mind, I wasn't quite convinced.

About five weeks later, well into the school year, I was trying to do some homework on the weekend. Suddenly, I started to feel extremely tired. No matter how I tried, I just couldn't keep my eyes open. I decided to lie down for the rest of the afternoon. After a few hours, I still felt tired when I got up. I felt like I hadn't rested at all.

The following day, it finally appeared. The day my life really changed. I couldn't push myself out of bed. I felt so heavy, as if I was stuck to my bed. My entire body was in pain. It took me about ten minutes to push myself out of bed. I felt so weak. I had no strength at all. All the energy had been drained from my body. I couldn't stand up properly. I had trouble bending my legs – a terrifying feeling. I crawled out of my room to see my parents and told them how I was feeling. They were distraught. It felt like the first time I had collapsed in Year 8, only this time, I felt much worse.

After a couple of days, I still felt the same. We had stopped seeing the rheumatologist after that very confronting and terse visit at the end of 1990 when I was in Year 9. However, I had continued taking the anti-inflammatory medication he had prescribed. I was still having only limited success with this medication, with my hands still quite swollen and painful. Mum had been given some information about a group of doctors, GPs who practised naturopathy. Given that we had tried other paths in trying to determine the cause of my previous symptoms of fatigue and joint pain, my parents and I thought that seeing one of these doctors was worth a try. Mum made me an appointment to see one of these doctors the following day (looking back, I don't know if that was good or bad that we got an appointment so quickly!). We had to travel all the way down to an elite beachside suburb in Melbourne's south, well over an hour from our home. I remember feeling so exhausted from the car ride. When greeted by the doctor on our arrival, he was a bespectacled, greying, middle-aged man. Reasonably friendly and eager to help, he documented my previous and current symptoms, including all of the difficulties with my hands.

At that stage the naturopathic doctor wasn't open with suggestions as to what could be causing my symptoms, but he insisted that I have two blood tests and a food allergy test performed. Without any pathology results to guide him, he immediately prescribed a huge list of vitamins and minerals for me to take every day. Mega doses of vitamin C, B and E, numerous multivitamin and multimineral tablets, zinc, iron, gingko biloba, garlic and three different types of circulation tablets such as nicotine acid and prickly ash that aimed to improve blood flow in my hands. In addition to these, an anti-inflammatory medication called Adalat® was also prescribed. The role of Adalat was to relieve pain in my hands and to increase blood flow. The vitamin and mineral tablets were to strengthen my immune system in the hope of eliminating toxins from my body in order to diminish fatigue and restore good health. I must admit, I did freak out, as any fifteen-year-old would, at the number of tablets I was expected to take each day – twenty-eight tablets! The doctors' clinic was quite the set-up, with a specialist chemist nearby that stocked all of their recommended pills and foods. It appeared to be a thriving business. We left the chemist that day with bags of these vitamins, minerals and strange concoctions. I felt so much for my parents. Raising a family with three teenagers on a single income, the financial impact of not only the doctor's appointment itself but the purchase of all of these tablets would have been financially draining and another stress in an already worrying and challenging time for them.

Remarkably, after a couple of days of taking these vitamins and minerals, I started to feel much brighter and really well again. I had more energy and my aches and pains had eased considerably. It was like I had been cleansed. In retrospect, that is exactly what would have happened as taking all of those vitamins and minerals was like a detoxification of my body's ills. I still felt a little wobbly, but after much discussion, my parents and I agreed that returning to school was worth a try. I wasn't that keen but realised that I had to see if I was truly improving and making progress.

So off I went, anxious but hopeful that I would be okay. After the first two periods of my first day back, I started to feel really tired and slow. I wasn't doing any class work. I just sat there in a daze, returning to my dream state of gazing out of the window. By recess, I made the decision to stay at school for another two periods to see if I would feel any better. I didn't – I felt worse. I remember having a double period of Art class. Our Art teacher was absent, so we had replacement teachers. I sat with my head in my hands for the double period. Not one of these teachers even noticed.

I made it to lunchtime at school and decided that I needed to go home. Mum didn't drive and Dad was at work, so I asked my home group teacher if he was available to drive me home. I had located him in the teachers' staff room. He was happy to drive me home, but I had to wait a minute. He was a kind and supportive teacher and aware of my health issues. I rang Mum from the school phone to let her know that my home group teacher was going to drive me home as soon as possible. Well, a minute turned into minutes and more minutes and at one stage whilst sitting outside the staffroom, I could see my home group teacher munching down on a yummy meat pie. Driving me home anytime soon was not looking good!

It was nearing the end of lunchtime and I was still waiting. I was starting to feel very agitated. I just wanted to go home. I had asked a teacher to check for me to see if my home group teacher was ready to take me. This teacher could not find him. Feeling forgotten, feeling frustrated and feeling so tired and desperate to leave, I made the decision to start walking home by myself. It was a ten to fifteen-minute walk from school to my house, but that day it took much, much longer than fifteen minutes. Honestly, I don't know how I managed to get home safely. I was nearly hit by a car crossing a very busy road. Fatigue was setting in and my ability to judge the mobility and speed of cars was limited. With every step I took, my muscles started to ache and I couldn't walk properly. I had no strength to support myself. I felt like a rag doll – floppy and weak. When I finally turned into my driveway, I was nearly crawling. Mum had been waiting for me at the front door, fraught with worry as it had taken me so long to arrive home. When she saw me, she burst into tears. So did I. I felt all the energy leave my body and collapsed into the hallway – I was overcome with relief that I had made it home.

* * *

I spent the next six weeks in bed. It was March 1991, and I remember not feeling much worry at that time because I was so sick. I didn't think much of anything. I slept and slept and slept, even when in pain. I started to lose large clumps of hair and lose more weight. When out of bed, I dragged myself around with the use of a walking stick. I lived in my pyjamas and dressing gown. I didn't have the strength to bathe myself, so Mum became my primary carer. In addition to these symptoms I was experiencing, a myriad of other symptoms started to appear at this time such as a chronic low-grade fever, severe headaches, mental confusion, bouts of insomnia, rashes and dandruff on my scalp, bouts of Candida infections such as vaginal thrush and a nasty lower pelvic rash.

During the follow-up visit to the naturopathic doctor at this time, the food allergy tests had arrived and they were not good. It seemed that I was allergic to wheat, yeast, dairy, eggs, lamb, capsicum and tomatoes. I was instructed to stop eating all of these foods immediately. The worst news was the ban on chocolate. Chocolate! It was no good for my blood circulation problems. A Candida infection in my bowel was present but blood tests showed that everything in my body appeared to be working well.

Whilst pathology tests continued to indicate that I was in apparent good health, given my food allergies and excessive fatigue, the naturopathy doctor diagnosed me with chronic fatigue syndrome. The condition is also known as M.E., which stands for myalgic encephalomyelitis. M.E. is a disorder characterised by extreme fatigue that can't be explained by any underlying medical condition. The fatigue may worsen with physical or mental activity but doesn't improve with rest. Diagnosis of this condition is based on clinical symptoms, not pathology as at that time (and still to this day) there was no definitive test available to diagnose M.E. more conclusively.[1]

This news was a lot to digest. Whilst the majority of symptoms I was experiencing were indicative of chronic fatigue syndrome, the blood circulation issues in my hands were still a concern. These symptoms were the major anomaly in this M.E. diagnosis. They didn't fit the profile of this condition at all. My parents and I felt a little relieved that we had a name that was more definitive in this journey to diagnose my symptoms, but we still felt apprehensive that we had found the complete answer. We decided to continue seeing the naturopathic doctor and monitor how I would respond to changes in my diet and the continued regime of the myriad of vitamin and mineral tablets, and if any improvements occurred.

My daily diet of breakfast and lunch consisted of yeast-free and wheat-free rolls, bread or pita bread. Back in the nineties, gluten-free and yeast-free products were extremely expensive and difficult to find. Carrot, alfalfa sprouts and sardines were recommended as substitute fillings for the foods such as tomatoes that I was no longer able to eat in sandwiches. Soy milk was the replacement for the dairy foods that I could no longer have. Dinner time wasn't as disrupted, only when pasta or dairy-based foods featured. I remember it being a monotonous diet; limited, bland

and difficult to digest. It didn't give me the much-needed joy that would have helped combat my fatigue and pain, that's for sure!

The anti-inflammatory medication Adalat that had been prescribed by the naturopathic doctor was not making any difference in relieving the pain in my hands. It was meant to improve the circulation of blood in my hands, but they were still cold and painful. The impact of taking the additional medication of prickly ash and nicotine acid was a mystery. The naturopathic doctor recommended that I double the dose of Adalat to see if this improved my pain. Within days, I started to feel more lethargic and very dizzy. Mum was worried so she took me to my local and trusted chemist for his opinion on the medication. He took my blood pressure and found it alarmingly low. The chemist advised me to stop taking the medication immediately. He also advised against taking the nicotine acid and especially the prickly ash. He said that this was a dangerous drug, particularly for someone of my age. Thankfully, my dizziness ceased and my lethargy improved slightly after ceasing Adalat.

The medication issue was at the cusp of about three months of this naturopathy regime and my parents were very concerned that the naturopathic doctor was not the best person to be treating me. Concerned about my response to taking the double dose of Adalat and the chemist's advice against taking the prickly ash and nicotine acid, Mum phoned the naturopathic doctor to inform him of the side effects I'd experienced. The doctor became very defensive and the conversation soon escalated to the point where Mum informed him that I would not be his patient anymore.

This was the right decision. Within the short time of seeing the naturopathic doctor, it felt as though he was not 100% sure about his diagnosis of M.E. and that the medications he prescribed were more like an experiment to see if my symptoms improved. We never felt that he was confident in what he prescribed, as he was not able to reassure us that the improvement in my symptoms was likely to occur. To this day, there is no singular pathology test that can accurately diagnose M.E. This made it very hard for us to fully accept that this was in fact the correct diagnosis of my symptoms.

My parents eased me off the vitamin and mineral regime and slowly reintroduced all of the foods I had stopped eating back into my daily diet. I did not display any obvious symptoms of food allergy such as gastrointestinal problems. When I began eating wheat and yeast products like bread and pasta again, I felt fine, so we figured I wasn't truly allergic as diagnosed. I stopped taking the Adalat and my dizziness and light-headedness improved.

I continued resting and hoping. Hoping that one day soon, the true reason for what was ailing me would emerge. That life would become brighter. Effortless. Simple. I kept on hoping.

Chapter Four

What are Family and Friends For?

The feeling of being 'in limbo' returned once more. Once again, there was no certainty about what was wrong with me. The well-worn path of visiting doctor after doctor was wearing me out. To not have definitive answers over such a long period of time was impacting on my spirit. I started to question the severity of my pain and wondered if I was really as sick as I felt.

Thankfully, self-doubt never turned to a depressed state. I just felt sad. Sad that the medical profession had not appraised my symptoms as urgent. I was never whisked into the hospital and given immediate attention when my symptoms became worse and more pronounced. Why wasn't anyone shouting, 'We must find out what is wrong with this poor girl and we will not stop until we do!' Where was my advocate in this medical world? Where was my crusader? No one appeared truly moved by my plight. No one was perplexed enough to say yes, all pathology indicates that she is healthy and well but there is something seriously wrong if she has no strength, no energy, is constantly fatigued, can't walk unaided, is experiencing joint and muscle pain, has poor circulation, is dizzy, is losing clumps of hair and is losing weight at an alarming rate. Finding the answer to my suffering just didn't feel like a priority in this medical world.

I couldn't help but feel very frustrated. Not long before I collapsed at the beginning of Year 10, a friend of mine from school developed joint pain and fatigue over the summer holidays. He was immediately admitted into the Royal Children's Hospital and rigorously screened and tested for all types of possible causes of his symptoms. He was not released from the hospital until they found out what was wrong with him. Reactive arthritis was the diagnosis and thankfully, with treatment and time, his symptoms improved and he returned to school not long after his short stay in the hospital.

Why was his experience so different from mine? It seemed that his suffering was made a priority. His account of the symptoms and pain he was experiencing were never challenged or doubted by the doctors who attended to him. Suffering from joint pain and fatigue, he was never scrutinised by a psychologist to see if there was an underlying emotional cause to his pain. He was never made to feel that he was not as sick as he felt. He was never made to doubt himself. His medical experience was the complete opposite to mine.

When my thoughts would drift to my experience and what was happening to me, I couldn't help but reflect on how similar our symptoms were but how different the medical response. I couldn't help but feel extremely angry by the way doctors had played down the severity of my pain and suffering, subjecting me to endless consultations, whereby I was told that what I was experiencing wasn't that bad. In stark contrast, my friend was taken seriously, genuinely cared for and made to feel that all efforts would be made to find the solution to his pain as soon as possible.

Why was there such disparity in the medical response to us as two young people with similar symptoms? The only possible reason I could think of was gender. I was a teenage girl; he, a teenage boy. I envisaged that teenage girls who lose weight, become fatigued and work hard at school would be pigeon-holed by doctors as 'anorexic', 'depressed' or 'perfectionists', and therefore, an emotional or mental health focus was the likely cause of these physical symptoms. Teenage boys who experienced similar symptoms would be taken more seriously, particularly if they have never experienced fatigue or joint pain before. They were less likely to have an eating disorder or to be overly studious at school. Therefore, something must be seriously wrong and finding the answer was a priority.

* * *

Being at home during this time was a lonely and isolating experience. Even though I had Mum with me during the day, I was yearning to be at school and amongst friends and peers. I felt forgotten – left behind. Friends stopped calling, stopped writing and stopped visiting. Each day, I would peer out of my lounge room window, rugged up in my long, pale blue dressing gown and slippers, watching the kids come home from school, wondering if anyone would stop to think of me and visit. I would think about the things I was missing. Sixteenth birthday parties and sleepovers, school excursions, the Year 10 camp to Tasmania, who was going out with who, the pranks and laughter of classroom silliness … the fun I was missing out on.

I would sleep in most days and Mum would help me to get out of bed. When I woke, I never ever felt refreshed. I felt so heavy, as if I hadn't slept at all. Mum would help me out of bed and to the kitchen table. Eating took much effort. I was very laboured with my breathing, so consuming each bite took time. Once I was finished, Mum would help me sit down on a plastic stool in the shower and wash me. I didn't have the strength to hold my arms up or dry my hair, so Mum would do that for me too. It would take at least an hour. It was a physically demanding job for her. An emotional one too, as clumps of my hair would tangle up in her hands and block the shower drain. It broke her heart to see me fading away like that, with no improvement in sight.

I used a walking stick to move around the house and literally take one step at a time. Then I would go back to bed. It was exhausting. It was such a worrying time for Mum and Dad, particularly in the night if I needed to go to the toilet. One night, I got out of bed on my own but by the time I made it inside the toilet, I had fainted. The noise gave Mum and Dad an awful fright, and they had much difficulty waking me up and getting me out of the toilet as I had somehow fallen down, half in the toilet and half out!

Around midday each day, the education I was missing out on was replaced by the school of Phil Donahue. The Donahue show was a daily American talk show and it featured many interesting topics that kept my mind a little more active. My parents had rigged up their small black and white bedroom television to sit at the edge of my desk for me to watch in bed. I shared a room with my sister and she loved it, as it sat right in front of her bed! Watching telly helped me pass the time as I didn't have the concentration nor the inclination to read. Every now and then I would try to read when I felt like trying to see if it would make a difference, but my eyes would glaze over the words and anything I read made little sense.

Mum tried everything to keep me optimistic. In an era when terms like 'mindfulness' were not being bandied about, Mum was ahead of her time, posting positive affirmations and pictures of vibrant, healthy people around my bedroom. They were symbols of hope and a reminder to stay focused on looking forward. I found them comforting. As I lay in bed looking around my room, I would linger on these images and genuinely feel hopeful that one day soon the answers to my plight would reveal themselves and that everything would be alright – that I was going to be alright.

Mum, Dad, my sister Rebecca and brother Ross were primarily the only people I was interacting with. They were my strength and my comfort – my everything. It was challenging for Dad. Raised in Darwin, he moved to Melbourne at the age of twenty to complete his studies in becoming a draftsman. He met Mum and stayed in Melbourne, raising his family and eventually working as a draftsman and project manager at Melbourne Airport for many years. His parents had passed away when I was a child, and his brothers and sisters were living in other parts of Australia, busy raising their families. Support from his side of the family was minimal due to these geographical distances.

Additionally, many of my friends, family and neighbours changed and stopped caring about me. It was devastating. At a time when my family and I needed much love and support, our hearts were breaking from the seemingly cold and callous way people we loved and cherished were treating us – or treating me specifically. I could just cope with the fading visits and lost friendships, but seeing the way family, friends and neighbours treated my parents was just awful and extremely painful for me to watch. They had enough to worry about. They didn't need any more disappointment. It was hard enough that the medical world was offering them limited support. To have loved ones not offer to help or to offer acts of kindness and compassion felt very cruel.

What are Family and Friends For?

* * *

One of the first moments when I felt a shift in how loved ones were responding to my plight was during a visit from my granny (Mum's mother) and uncle (partner of my aunty, Mum's sister). Granny lived in the country, the town of Bacchus March, and was visiting Melbourne, staying with my aunty and uncle. She had been speaking regularly with Mum about my health and was concerned that the doctors couldn't find the answer to what was ailing me. At times, these conversations were very stressful for Mum, as granny would scrutinise the care that Mum and Dad were giving me. She was very critical of their efforts. Mum would get off the phone feeling frustrated that she did not have her mother's full understanding that there was nothing anyone could do at that time that would provide the answers we were all so desperately seeking. She didn't need to be questioned or judged. She needed someone to listen to her and to offer her comfort and words of solace. She just needed her mum.

My granny and uncle wanted to visit us to give Mum a fortieth birthday present on behalf of my aunty, who was too busy at the time to visit herself. Upon their arrival, I gathered my strength to get up out of bed and entered the lounge room where they were seated with Mum. As I hobbled into the room, clutching my walking stick, I could see the shock on my granny's and uncle's faces. It was a long, five-minute walk to the sofa. I had to place the walking stick in front of me and drag my legs to follow. I'm sure it was a sorry sight. They both looked extremely uncomfortable. The realisation that I was this sick was clearly dawning on them. My granny was hesitant to kiss or embrace me. I felt contagious.

What followed was devastating for Mum. In a phone call the next day after their visit, my granny bluntly ordered Mum to have me anointed by a priest. She was clearly affected by the severity of my illness, but instead of offering my mum comforting or compassionate words, she felt that the only way to cure me was using religion. A terse discussion ensued, with Mum trying to convince my granny that being anointed by a priest was not what I needed. Offended and exasperated, Mum found an excuse to quickly get off the phone.

Two months followed and there was no contact from my granny or aunty to see how I was progressing. In the end, Dad rang my aunty to enquire about my granny and to calmly let them know that Mum and I were both hurt by their abrupt silence and neglect. All my aunty could say was that both she and my granny had been 'naughty'. Not long after this conversation, a book and cards from my aunty and granny arrived in the mail. I did not wish to receive them, as I felt that they had only been sent because Dad had prompted them to do so.

Another two months passed and still no contact from my granny or aunty. Were they afraid to visit? Maybe they were scared of catching what I was suffering from, given that the doctors did not know what was ailing me. I found their behaviour quite distressing and remember frequently asking Mum, 'Why? What have I done?' I was already socially isolated and without regular contact from school friends. To have members of my own family cast me aside like this was so hurtful, not to mention a detriment to my health. To combat my physical symptoms, I needed to stay positive and keep my spirit as strong as possible. Their neglect was not helping me at all. It made Mum extremely sad and upset too.

Upon much reflection, her distance wasn't a complete surprise to me. My granny was a devout Catholic and very strict in the upbringing of her four children. At times, a very jealous and controlling person – always critical of my mother's actions. Mum was the youngest and she felt that granny was the hardest on her out of the four children. As Mum was a homemaker, my granny expected Mum to be at the end of the phone whenever she rang. If Mum didn't answer, she would be grilled and scrutinised. Little affection was shown to her children. Kisses, hugs and expressions of 'I love you' did not come naturally, if at all.

In contrast to her parenting skills, my granny was more loving, kind and much-valued within her community. She regularly frequented her local church and had special roles in many undertakings, including ironing the priest's shirts. It appeared that she had more love to give to the parish, her friends and neighbours than members of her own family. She was always the first to comfort those who were ill, with the utmost care. Acts of kindness such as cards, cakes and home visits were always given. She was well known in her community for her compassion. She was praised and adored. But when it came to illness in her own family, the complete opposite was her response. It seemed that being sick was frowned upon – a weakness that was only to befall others, for her family needed to appear healthy and strong.

My granny's relationship with my brother, sister and me was always kind but it also felt emotionally distant. We were given treats when we visited her home but we also needed to meet her strict expectations. She would be easily crossed and annoyed if we made too much noise. It was difficult to just be children when in her company. Out of the three of us, I did not look like my brother or sister at all. They have pale skin and blonde, sandy hair and are clearly descendants of Mum and my granny's side of the family, whereas I had the dark looks of my father – thick, brown hair, brown eyes and dark, olive skin. My physical appearance stood out and I was always being asked which part of Italy I was from! It was hard enough growing up having people at school say to Mum when I was with her, 'And who is this girl then?' When Mum replied that I was her daughter, the 'oohs' and 'aahs' that followed would make me feel like an outcast. I didn't like the special attention, and being spoken about like this made feel uncomfortable and self-conscious.

My granny treated me a little like the school's mums – differently from my brother and sister as we grew up. The differences were always subtle. I was never fussed over like they were. I remember one day when I was around twelve years old, we were celebrating my granny's eightieth birthday. She proudly introduced the three of us to her parish priest, 'This is my grandson, Ross, this is my granddaughter Rebecca, and this is Rachel Lea.' I've never forgotten those words. During that moment, shocked and upset as I was, it became clear how she truly felt about me. I didn't represent her family. I didn't belong.

During this time of angst between my aunty, my granny and parents, I had an appointment with a paediatric psychiatrist visiting the Royal Children's Hospital from England. After assessing my situation, he reported that my mental health was fine and he was satisfied that I was coping well. Mum enquired as to how she should cope with her mum and sister and all of the stress they were causing. The psychiatrist told my Mum that her first duty was to her own family and that she didn't owe her mum and sister anything. He suggested that Mum cease communication with them at this time, as she had enough on her plate to deal with.

Mum wrote a letter to both of them, explaining that she was taking a break from them for now. She had to put all of her energy into caring for me and our family and did not have time for their lack of support. Mum did not forbid them from contacting Dad, Ross, Rebecca or me. Personally, I did not want anything to do with them. My heart had become too sore from their lack of care for me.

Astonishingly, when my sixteenth birthday came around, my aunty sent me gifts and a birthday card. Written in the birthday card was a shocking message, accusing me of slowly killing my granny as I had not been in contact with her. It was just awful to receive this card and read such an appalling accusation. It was beyond comprehension. I was extremely upset. My only crime was being sick. Dad, furious and fed up, sent a letter to my aunty, telling her to leave Mum and me alone.

Not long after, defying Dad's request of no correspondence, Mum received a letter from my aunty. It was full of inane and trivial stories of her recent trip to Sydney. She wrote as though there was nothing wrong, as though she hadn't written those cruel words to me at all. In the conclusion, she made the comment, 'I will visit Rachel when she is all better again.' Her love for me as her niece was clearly conditional. My aunty would be waiting a very, very long time as I was not going to get better anytime soon. Whilst distressing to process these words, it was another validation that my resolve to not communicate with either my aunty or my granny was more than okay.

Mum responded to this letter by outlining in great detail all of the hardship that she and Dad were going through with me. She made it clear how my aunty's behaviour had affected the whole family. Mum stated that if she or my granny wanted to know how I was progressing, they could contact Dad.

My granny and my aunty never reached out to Dad to see how I was progressing or to see how Mum was coping. The silence would last eight long years. It was devastating for Mum. It seemed that a challenging event like my illness exposed their hearts and minds in a way that she hadn't seen before. Had they changed or was this who they really were all along? I feared the latter.

While we didn't have my granny's or my aunty's support during that difficult time, as a family, we had each other. Mum and Dad sought much comfort in each other and did their best to overcome this heartbreak and focus their energy on taking care of their children, particularly me. The strength that this required was often tested but, ultimately, the knowledge that we as a family did not need any undue stress from uncaring family members such as my granny and my aunty would centre us as a family unit and give us the perspective we needed. For being true to ourselves was the shining light that we needed to get through the darkness of not knowing what was to come.

* * *

Many years later, when my granny was dying, Mum and my aunty reunited. What happened during that time of absence in each other's lives has never been spoken of since, as they simply focused on taking care of my granny in her final days. I visited my granny on her death bed for the first time since all of those years ago when my illness caused this heartbreaking family conflict. Forgiveness was in my heart and still is. I don't know and will never know why she did not embrace me with more tolerance and compassion during my time of need. I simply made peace with what had happened and have tried my hardest since to let it go. I have seen my aunty at the occasional family event over the years, but I have made it clear that I do not wish to resume a relationship with her. She has never apologised to me nor made any efforts to heal what was broken all of those years ago.

Chapter Five

Fighting Back with Scrabble and Cups of Tea

Each day continued to feel like Groundhog Day; the same tasks played out on repeat. Sleep, wake up, eat, shower, rest, eat, rest, eat, sleep. Repeat. I wondered, how long was I going to live like this? Was I ever going to be well enough to attend school again? What if I had a disease that was not curable? Was I going to die? There was so much time for my mind to drift and linger in fear and uncertainty. Staying positive and hopeful was a challenge when my mind was overwhelmed with worries like these.

With no diagnosis in sight, I needed to find a way to fight back. I needed to keep my spirit strong. But how do you fight back when you don't even know what you are fighting? Looking back now, I can see how easy it would have been to plummet into a state of complete hopelessness, to wallow in my suffering and not look ahead with any hope for brighter days.

Thankfully, I had parents who gave me the gift of focusing on what I was able to do, and they would guide me out of the sad state of pondering on what I couldn't do. They reminded me that by simply getting through each day, I was making progress. Their encouragement was everything to me and I would find much comfort in realising the small achievements I was able to make. It was not in my nature to feel slighted or sorry for myself (well, I had my moments!) Somehow, at the tender age of sixteen, I knew that I was not in control of my life – that no one is. What I was experiencing could happen to anyone, at any time. I didn't realise just how mature and insightful I was during this time. In retrospect, I believe these qualities gave me much strength and perspective. The ability to feel gratitude in every step I made was empowering. I began to truly appreciate how fortunate I really was, despite experiencing the anguish of an unknown future.

Despite my feelings of despair, I knew that keeping my spirit strong required more peace and positivity in each day. For that to happen, I needed to have greater purpose. If my physical symptoms were to have any chance of improving, I had to manage my pain with greater mental strength. Simply, I needed more courage and more faith that, no matter what the outcome, I was going to be okay.

Mum and I began to work on creating new goals that I could work towards achieving. My first big goal was to improve my ability to walk longer distances. Each day, we would name destination points that I would try and walk towards. Other than moving around the house with my walking stick, the front porch was the first destination point outside the house that I was strong enough to walk to. For a long time, this was as far as I could walk. I was not strong enough to walk down the porch steps, so when I was able to do this, it was literally a step forward. It was at least five steps from the bottom of the porch steps to reach the prickle bush situated halfway down the driveway – another destination point to conquer. When I was able to get this far, the letterbox at the end of the driveway became my next target. Then my neighbour's letterbox, then her neighbour's letterbox and so on.

The ultimate destination was the top of the court where I lived. The distance was walking past four houses on the right side of our house. It took me many months to get there, walking stick in hand, but when I finally stood at this juncture, I was quite emotional. My body had become so deconditioned due to my prolonged sedentary state. Physical activity such as this was critical in strengthening my muscle mass, improving my lung capacity and boosting my spirits. My smile truly widened with every step forward I was able to make as I felt more empowered and hopeful.

In addition to these walking goals, I began daily meditation. Mum accessed some beautiful relaxation tapes that I would listen to each day. I used all of the classic meditative mantras such as imagining and breathing in bright lights of different colours, directing the breath to all parts of the body. I found meditating really helpful and, over time, I started to feel slightly energised from this practice. Affirmations of positivity continued to be posted around my room, and I made more effort to read them over and over and absorb their healing energy.

I'd like to think that if I was experiencing the symptoms I had back then in the nineties today, the medical profession would take a broader, more holistic, view in recommending alternative practices such as relaxation and meditation techniques in trying to help ease my pain and find a way forward for me, despite not knowing the actual cause of my ailing health. I was really left to languish by the medical profession back then, simply because all of the pathology tests stated that I was fine – no illness here. It makes me more emotional thinking back to this time and the resolve my parents had in trying to help ease my pain and keep my attitude positive and strong, despite such uncertainty. Their love and dedication in taking care of me has gone unrecognised by many, particularly during that time, and in retrospect, I feel much sadness about that.

* * *

With walking goals and meditation added to my daily rituals, the issue of my education needed attention too. With Mum's proactive research, she discovered that I was entitled to receive visits from a visiting teachers' service that was offered by the Department of Education. I started receiving visits from the visiting teacher during the middle of 1991. I was very nervous before her first visit. My concentration was very poor and I was anxious about whatever task she had in store for me. When she arrived, it was like a huge burst of energy blew through the door. She was a very tall, large lady in her late forties with a loud, booming voice. She laughed easily and reassured me that our time together would not be too serious. Her name was Jackie and she was a retired primary school teacher. Her work as a visiting teacher involved working as a tutor for sick and disabled children in their homes.

At this time, my school had not sent any work for me to complete at home. I was not capable of reading much so it would have been a pointless task. As I was struggling to concentrate and to recognise and decipher the meaning of key words, Jackie, Mum and I would play Scrabble during our sessions together. My cognitive skills were so poor, I had difficulty spelling three-letter words. I knew that I had to work hard at even a simple game like Scrabble if I was to regain these skills.

Jackie's major goal was to help me to remember how to spell and recognise words in a fun way. When it was my turn during the game, I would often pause and ponder on which word to place down. I was very slow at making decisions but this was of much benefit to Mum and Jackie, as they were able to continue chatting and sipping their cups of tea. The words I could place on the Scrabble board were not brilliant by any means but the cognitive muscles in my brain were being put to work, which was a major step forward for me. Jackie would visit our home two-to-three times a week and we would play Scrabble during each visit. Over time, I started to feel more confident and capable with my spelling and word association, but I was quite exhausted after each of these sessions, not to mention being a little sick of Scrabble!

Jackie's visits proved to be very beneficial for Mum as well. Mum was also very isolated from taking care of me with limited support from her family or friends, so it was lovely for Mum to have a supportive person to talk to and socialise with. They shared many cups of tea together and bonded over the experiences of motherhood and the difficulties in receiving the support needed from the medical profession.

Jackie was also a terrific support as a liaison between me and the teachers from school. She became my advocate and set up a teacher support group for me – the first ever support group for a sick student in the history of my secondary school. When my concentration and strength improved to a point where I was ready to tackle reading books and completing small written tasks, Jackie arranged a meeting of all of my Year 10 teachers and informed them of my current progress. She arranged for a small amount of schoolwork, mainly English, to be organised for me to start completing at home at my own pace. My English teacher proved to be a great support during this time and would sometimes call in at home to collect work that I had completed and to say hello. She even arranged for students in my English class to write me letters of greetings and well wishes. It lifted my spirits tremendously.

I started to feel more connected to the outside world, which was integral in helping me to persevere through all of the uncertainty at this time. I was finally making gains in my physical strength, and to see my concentration improving too, made me feel much happier and brighter within myself. Maybe I would return to school one day soon after all.

Chapter Six

Is It Lupus?

As I continued to make progress with my daily walking tasks and Scrabble visits from Jackie, the issue of finding answers to the true cause of my symptoms was still at the forefront of every day. As I had ceased seeing the naturopathic GP, my parents wondered what to do next. I still had a valid referral to see the paediatric rheumatologist at the Royal Children's Hospital, so my parents made an appointment to see him. We were interested in his professional opinion on our experience with the naturopathic GP and his diagnosis of chronic fatigue syndrome, or M.E.

Thankfully, we didn't have to wait too long to see him. My parents filled him in with what had been happening since our last visit with him, which was about eighteen months ago. Mum asked him about the possibility of me having M.E. and whether the naturopathic GP was on the right track with his diagnosis. The rheumatologist gave his honest opinion that he was not sure, as he had no expertise in the appraisal of M.E. symptoms. He referred me to a paediatrician at the Royal Children's Hospital, who specialised in M.E., in the hope that this doctor may be able to provide more definitive answers.

The rheumatologist was also quite concerned with the deterioration of my hands since our last appointment. He suggested that I continue taking the anti-inflammatory medication called Voltaren® (which was prescribed by the previous rheumatologist I had been seeing). He also booked me in for some aquatic physiotherapy to be undertaken again at the Royal Children's Hospital. He felt that I could benefit from completing some gentle exercises with my hands in water.

Whilst waiting to see the paediatrician, my parents and I began our regular visits to the Royal Children's Hospital to complete my hydrotherapy. I had to immerse my hands in a large container of temperature-regulated water and complete a range of fine motor skill tasks with objects such as squishy balls to strengthen my hands' movement. Completing these tasks felt a bit weird, but I felt like, finally, more action was being taken, which made me feel like the medical profession was working a little harder in trying to figure out was wrong with me.

The appointment for the paediatrician finally came around. Another new doctor, another long account of my medical journey so far. Thankfully, my parents and I were becoming quite proficient in summing up my symptoms and medical history during the many doctors' consultations we had experienced. The paediatrician was a lovely lady. Soft-spoken, fair-haired and in her late forties, she listened intently to the myriad of symptoms from which I had been suffering. On answering the question as to whether I had M.E., she felt that the symptoms I had suffered from did not match the criteria used to diagnose the condition. Prior to the consultation, I had done some blood and urine tests for the paediatrician. The ESR (Erythrocyte Sedimentation Rate) blood test was slightly elevated, suggesting inflammation in my body. This was a significant breakthrough compared with the previous blood tests I had completed, all of which indicated that there was no presence of a virus or disease. The new test results indicated that something more definitive was on the horizon – more hope that a diagnosis could possibly be made soon.

As I had not experienced a virus prior to the onset of my symptoms, the paediatrician did not believe that I had M.E. In most cases, sufferers of the condition experience a flu or virus that leaves them with debilitating fatigue and a myriad of symptoms. She wanted to keep an eye on the slight changes in my blood tests and asked to see me for a follow up visit a few weeks later, with more blood tests to be performed. She wished to continue seeing me to help monitor my progress and to help me return to school.

What a positive visit this was. Maybe, a possible answer to my suffering was not far away. Not to mention that the paediatrician was personable, understanding, caring and prepared to help us find out what was wrong with me. Furthermore, she wanted to help me get back to school – a massive step forward. The care we had received from the rheumatologist and the paediatrician was excellent, and I felt truly cared for by the medical team at the Royal Children's Hospital.

* * *

With my spirits higher, I continued to complete more and more schoolwork from home. My energy was improving and I felt much stronger. I was able to walk longer distances without the aid of my walking stick, which was a wonderful achievement. I could even shower by myself and wash my own hair! However, I still needed to sleep during the day, mainly in the afternoons.

During my follow-up appointment with the paediatrician, she felt that it would be a good idea for me to make visits to school so that I could reconnect socially with my friends and classmates. She did not want me to worry about being an active student in the class. She simply wanted me to be in the classroom; to sit amongst my classmates, observe my teachers and be in the environment that I had been isolated from for so long.

As it was the end of the school year by this stage, it was a good time to visit school. My visits from Jackie became more focused on my return to school and making sure that I had what I needed to make my integration back into the classroom as smooth and stress-free as possible. The prospect of returning to school was both scary and exciting. I had not seen many people from school during my year-long absence and the thought of just arriving to class one day made me very anxious. Everyone would be gawking at me! What would I say? Where would I sit? I absolutely hated being the centre of attention. I would have to overcome all of my anxiety and just take it one step at a time.

Jackie had arranged for a teacher support group meeting to discuss the nature of my return visits to school. Another new experience – sitting in a room with all of my teachers at the same time to discuss me. The prospect of this meeting felt strange, as I had only spent a short time in their classes. It would also be the first time I had visited school after being absent for most of the year. I knew that it would be overwhelming to be in this environment again. I needed to take a deep breath and try not to worry too much.

Mum, Jackie, all of my Year 10 subject teachers and I met in a fancy conference room at school. Jackie ran the meeting, informing my teachers of my health issues, what I was capable of completing work-wise and that the purpose of my visits to their classes was to simply sit and observe. If I felt well enough to complete work, I could but I was not expected to at this time. Most of my teachers seemed positive and supportive of this arrangement (there were a couple of teachers who looked bored and were non-responsive during the meeting!) The next step for me would be to walk back into the classroom, find the courage to overcome my shyness and face my peers.

* * *

When the time came for my first day back, I found it quite emotional. Feelings of apprehension, fear and excitement were fluttering in my heart and mind. Whilst I was looking forward to seeing my friends and classmates, I also felt unsure about the ease in which I would slip back into being a part of my peer group. I was still feeling quite hurt and disappointed that I had been forgotten by my friends. Not being able to verbalise this to them was tough. During my absence from school, the one thing I struggled with the most was that whilst there was an initial expression of care at the beginning of my illness, my friends and classmates did not even wonder how I was progressing. They didn't wish to know if I was even getting better. It felt as though it was 'outta sight, outta mind' and life as a sixteen-year-old would have continued to open up for them. Their kinship with one another would have grown stronger. They had a year of rolling eyes with one another when their teachers were giving them grief. A year of discovering themselves, crafting the direction life after school would take them. A year of deeper friendships, shared interests, fun and possibly romance. A year of maturity that I was not going to match.

However, when I reflected more deeply, maybe I was the one that had experienced more growth and maturity than they had. Just because I was unable to participate in the social world of an average sixteen-year-old at school or experience the milestones that they had, it didn't mean that I was behind. If anything, I had moved forward. I was probably going to return to school a completely different person to the one they knew before my absence. I was going to be more serious. For every day I was able to be well enough to attend school would mean so much more to me than ever before. The appreciation I would have for how far I had progressed, from being completely bedridden, to fighting back on minimal medication and without an official diagnosis, being able to walk with more ease, greater strength and less pain, would shape me into a young woman with more resolve to make the most of each day. The gratitude I would feel for simply being able to participate in the world would be savoured. I was definitely going to be different from my peers – and significantly so.

In accepting that none of us know what will greet us each day, the onus was going to be on me to truly make each day count. I now had an awareness of the fragility of life that I would otherwise not have had at all if this illness hadn't struck me down at this time in my life. Therefore, I knew that before I stepped back into the classroom, I was going to find it hard to share the experiences of my friends and to fit in.

The truth was that I didn't have close friends, let alone a best friend. All of my friends from primary school went to a different secondary school, which made me quite sad and lonely when I began Year 7. Being absent at the end of Year 8 and on and off again in Year 9 had also made it difficult for me to create true and meaningful friendships. I was always a little bit different from everyone – too sensible and mature, which made it difficult to find other like-minded kindred spirits. Then, to be absent for most of Year 10? Well, I was completely out of the social loop now. It would be really difficult to find my place socially – this, I knew. I simply had to accept my experience for what it was and to let go of the unfairness of it all. I already had too much to rise above and I didn't need to add resentment to my list of battles.

The discussion of how I would travel to and from school was quite involved. Whilst my physical strength had improved, I was not capable of walking fifteen minutes to and from school. As Mum didn't drive and Dad was at work, we decided that Mum would push me to school in a wheelchair. As I was not staying at school for long, one or two periods at a time, Mum would be waiting at the school gate with the wheelchair, ready to push me all the way home when I finished. This was an onerous task for Mum, let alone the likely stares she would likely receive simply from pushing an empty wheelchair down the street! Mum had her own health battles, so this was a huge undertaking for her and a task that I am so very grateful for to this day.

Whilst I was not looking forward to being ostracised, I realised that on my return, any initial interest from my friends and classmates would hopefully be fleeting. Thankfully, it was. But it wasn't easy. Re-establishing friendship groups was very hard. As predicted, everyone was tightly bound in their own friendship groups. Most people were kind but there was the odd hurtful comment and ignorance to overcome. One boy called out to me, 'We heard you were dying.' The quickest retort I could come up with was, 'Gee, thanks for coming to say goodbye.' I just had to breathe deeply, stand taller and simply enjoy being at school.

The sensory overload of being back in a classroom was quite intense. I spent most of the time in a daze. Students and teachers would be talking but I would just stare at the whiteboard or out the window, detailing all that I had missed. I just couldn't believe I was actually sitting in class. I was out of my pyjamas, out of my bed and actually participating in the world. It felt joyful. It felt strange. But mostly, it felt normal. Listening to my teachers took much energy so one or two periods was more than enough at that stage. I would simply sit amongst the class and try to engage in what was happening but my efforts were minimal. I still had a long way to go in regard to being an active student.

***

Not long after my return to school, we had another support group meeting to discuss my future as a VCE student. VCE stands for Victorian Certificate of Education and is completed over the final two years of secondary school in the state of Victoria, Year 11 and Year 12. With the significant absences from school that I had from the end of Year 8 and most of Year 10, my ability to catch up on all that I had missed academically and socially felt quite overwhelming. I was unsure of what would become of me – unclear about what the expectations were going to be. After much discussion, thankfully, I was not expected to repeat Year 10. Being a serious, dedicated and high-performing student in my previous school years had paid off! The minimal amount of work I was able to complete at home toward the end of Year 10 also contributed to the decision that was made.

It was very gratifying to learn that my teachers held such praise and confidence in me and my ability to recommence school in Year 11 without completing Year 10. However, it was not going to be easy. Despite demonstrating the aptitude to cope with the demands of being in VCE, my absences had minimised the selection of subjects I could choose. The challenge would be selecting subjects that I enjoyed but also had every chance of succeeding in.

The question of how many VCE units to complete in Year 11 and Year 12 was also an issue. I was not well enough to have a full student load. The difficulty of not knowing what I was suffering from or if or when I would recover and become a full-time student again made these decisions very difficult to make. The most realistic solution was to complete my VCE over three years. I felt very anxious about this. I was already behind academically and socially, and the thought of sinking further behind my peers was upsetting. So, I found my voice at this meeting and I suggested that I complete the minimum number of units to satisfactorily complete VCE – which is sixteen units over two years. This equated to completing four subjects each semester. That way, I would be completing Year 11 and Year 12 with my peers and hopefully graduating with them too.

Nevertheless, it was not the ideal solution, as I would have to pass every single one of these sixteen units to satisfactorily pass my VCE. I could not fail one single subject, and I would need to perform extremely well in all of them in Year 12 if I wanted to achieve my dream of becoming a teacher. I needed to surpass a minimum score in order to be accepted into uni and study to become a teacher. This was a lot of pressure at an already trying and unclear time in my young life. I wanted to be given the opportunity to do it. I didn't think it was fair to rule me out before giving me a chance to even try.

Flash forward to the future, in my work as a VCE secondary school teacher, over time I became more sentimental and reflective in my teaching. I developed an acronym that is a reminder of this time in my life as an embattled VCE student. When I am marking student work, I write the acronym APPS on their work. It stands for 'Anything is possible, so with pride and perseverance, strive.' I created this acronym to give my students hope and to reinforce greater self-belief in their own capabilities that when they work hard and simply try, anything can happen. It has much personal meaning to me, as I fought for permission to be given the opportunity to complete my VCE according to the timeline that I thought was possible.

With more deliberation, it was agreed that I could complete my VCE in sixteen units. If my health deteriorated and I was not coping with the workload, I could then stretch it out and complete my VCE over three years. The decision to allow me to complete my VCE in this way gave me much hope and more control over the course my life was taking. It was important for my health too. Having experienced so much illness, which was completely out of my control, it felt good to be able to contribute to the direction of my future education.

* * *

By December 1991, I had continued to attend school when I was able. My parents and I were encouraged by the progress that I was making. I continued to see the paediatrician at the Royal Children's Hospital. During my visit before Christmas, the doctor had some serious news to share. The recent blood tests that had been performed indicated a significant change and that a possible diagnosis for my puzzling symptoms was imminent. My paediatrician felt that my blood test results were pointing towards a diagnosis of lupus – Systemic Lupus Erythematosus to be exact. She said that the professor of rheumatology who I had been previously seeing at the Royal Children's Hospital was more expert in assessing the possible changes that were occurring, so she referred me to see him immediately.

This news was profound. For the first time during these years of searching for a diagnosis, this was the first time a doctor was prepared to name the possible cause of my symptoms. My parents and I were aware of the significance of this disclosure. Whilst we were still waiting for the official confirmation, it was a massive step closer to finally knowing what was wrong with me.

Upon our return visit, the professor of rheumatology explained that my ESR and other inflammatory marker blood tests were slowly increasing. He agreed with the paediatrician that given the list of symptoms I had suffered from, such as debilitating fatigue, joint and muscle pain, the pathology was indicating that I was suffering from lupus. He advised me to look closely at my face each day during the summer holidays for signs of a red rash. A butterfly rash, to be precise. A butterfly rash is synonymous with having lupus. It is a red, raised rash that spreads across the nose and cheeks, emulating the shape of a butterfly, hence the name butterfly rash. If the rash appeared, it was most definitely lupus.

My parents and I left the children's hospital that day very quietly. A close family friend of ours suffered from lupus so we were well aware of the seriousness of this disease. We couldn't believe that after all of this time I could be suffering from a disease with which we were familiar.

It was both amazing and strange to think that the next step in my eventual diagnosis would be examining my face each and every day for a rash in the shape of a butterfly. A butterfly. A delicate, pretty and harmless creature that represented joy and freedom – the two aspects of my life that would be soon changed forever.

Chapter Seven

Well, It Is Lupus

The rheumatologist proved to be right. It happened a few weeks after our initial visit. I remember the day very clearly when I saw the butterfly rash appear on my face. It was a lovely sunny day and I was home, outside in the backyard. I started to feel a little hot and flushed so I decided to go inside. I was in the bathroom and I happened to look up at myself in the bathroom mirror. There it was, staring back at me, full blown and clearly defined. A red, raised butterfly rash.

I showed my parents, and as soon as they both took one look at me, we knew. We finally knew.

It was quite extraordinary that the rheumatologist's prediction of the butterfly rash appearing in a matter of weeks was so accurate. We made an appointment to see the rheumatologist, who upon hearing that the butterfly rash had appeared, wanted to see me immediately.

It was a momentous visit to see him. I remember that he looked both excited and worried. His eyes were shining with happiness for me. Happiness that after three years of experimental medicine, misdiagnosis, and not to mention doubt and extreme distress, I finally had a name for my condition. The rheumatologist sat directly in front of me, reached for my hands, looked into my eyes and proceeded to tell me the way forward. He said that I was going to be able to take a type of medication called corticosteroids (steroids) that would hopefully make me feel much better. If my symptoms did not improve from taking this medication, and if I did not notice a change in the fatigue and pain I was feeling, then it was not lupus. However, given that I had the butterfly rash, my history of symptoms, and an elevated ESR and other inflammatory markers in my pathology tests, he was extremely confident that it was lupus.

Despite the diagnosis of an incurable, potentially fatal disease, Mum, Dad and I walked out of the Royal Children's Hospital smiling and hugging each other. We had tears in our eyes too, but we were so relieved. We really did have a name. My suffering was legitimate. I was not imagining my symptoms. It was not in my head. I can't express in words the enormity of how that felt for me. Whilst I always knew that I was not responsible for making myself sick, after so many doctor's visits, so much discussion of what could be ailing me and so many comments during this time that my pain was not that bad or that it was self-induced, the relief was indescribable.

The plan was to take an extremely high dose of prednisolone, a commonly used type of corticosteroid in the treatment of lupus. I also had to continue taking the inflammatory medicine Voltaren to treat the pain in my hands. My parents and I headed straight to the hospital chemist and I took the prednisolone without trepidation. I was so excited to see what was going to happen.

Our appointment with the rheumatologist was in the morning, but later that day we were headed to the airport to see my aunty and uncle. They were transiting through Melbourne on their way home to Tasmania after holidaying in the mainland. When we arrived at the airport, I spotted the famous cricketer and broadcaster, Richie Benaud. He was walking through the turnstiles with his wife. Whilst exciting as it was to see someone famous, for some strange reason, I started laughing. And laughing. I just couldn't stop. In fact, I felt absolutely euphoric. I felt great. I started to feel lighter, with so much more energy. It was an amazing feeling. I was buzzing. It was like I had been a closed, droopy flower and, all of a sudden, my petals had begun to open to full bloom. The steroids were working! Whilst the sad diagnosis of lupus was hanging in the air, there was the renewed feeling that I was going to feel better by taking this medication. How joyous this was. This truly was a great day.

Chapter Eight

So, What Is Lupus?

So, what is lupus? To quote Professor Daniel J Wallace, systemic lupus erythematosus 'develops when the body becomes allergic to itself. In lupus, the body overacts to an unknown stimulus and makes too many antibodies, or proteins, directed against body tissue.'[2]

Specifically, lupus is a chronic autoimmune disease that, for unknown reasons, causes the immune system to attack any part of the body's own tissue and organs, including the joints, kidneys, heart, lungs, brain, blood or skin. Lupus can cause a wide variety of devastating symptoms. It can affect nearly every organ in the body with no predictability, causing widespread infections and inflammation.

A healthy immune system protects the body against viruses, bacteria and other foreign materials. With an autoimmune disease such as lupus, the immune system loses its ability to tell the difference between foreign substances and its own cells and tissue. The immune system then makes antibodies directed against 'itself', affecting each patient differently.

As lupus can affect so many different organs, a wide range of signs and symptoms can occur. These symptoms may come and go, and different symptoms may appear at different times during the course of the disease. The most common symptoms of lupus (which are the same for men and women) are:

- extreme fatigue (tiredness, no energy);
- headaches;
- painful or swollen joints;
- fever;
- anaemia (low numbers of red blood cells or haemoglobin, or total blood volume);
- swelling (oedema) in feet, legs, hands, and/or around the eyes;
- pain in the chest on deep breathing (pleurisy);
- butterfly-shaped rash across cheeks and nose;
- sun or light sensitivity (photosensitivity);
- hair loss;
- abnormal blood clotting;
- fingers turning white, red and/or blue when cold (known as Raynaud's phenomenon); and
- mouth or nose ulcers.[3]

Diagnosing lupus can be challenging, as there is not a single test that can definitively diagnose lupus. It can take months, sometimes years, to determine if someone is suffering from lupus. Doctors are likely to examine the combination of a person's symptoms, their medical history, family history and lab tests to diagnose lupus.[4]

As described earlier, the first symptoms of lupus that appeared for me were extremely cold hands, chilblains and then chronic pain in my hands. These symptoms were followed by muscle weakness, debilitating fatigue, pain in major joints, fever, skin rashes and headaches. Not long after, extreme weight loss and hair loss became more pronounced, along with the appearance of the butterfly rash on my face and sensitivity to the sun and UV rays. In the last thirty years, I have continued to suffer from these symptoms, but I have also experienced a few changes. During the first twenty years, the results from the frequent urine tests I completed, which aimed to examine how my kidneys were functioning, were perfect. However, over the latter ten years, my urine has shown traces of blood and protein, signs of possible changes in the kidneys. As a result, I have been seeing kidney specialists over the years to monitor the health of my kidneys. I have also been under the care of an excellent endocrinologist during the past few years, as I have developed large nodules in my thyroid. According to pathology, while these nodules are not signs of Hashimoto's disease that causes hypothyroidism, they are a sign that some type of thyroid disease or activity is occurring. It is proving very difficult to specifically diagnose.

Thankfully, at this time, all is well in my kidneys and a biopsy of a significant nodule in my thyroid is cancer-free, but it is a serious reminder that I must be extremely vigilant in recognising and reporting any changes that I notice in my body. Throughout the years, routine tests have always been performed to ensure that my major organs such as heart, lungs and kidneys, are always functioning well. Lupus Warriors, as we call ourselves, already have so many aspects of our health to worry about, we must also find the strength and courage to examine changes in our bodies, despite how confronting the prospect of more health issues may appear.

Systemic lupus erythematosus (also known as SLE), which causes inflammation in multiple organs and body systems, is the most common form of lupus. There are three other types of lupus. Firstly, discoid lupus erythematosus only affects the skin and is also known as cutaneous lupus. Secondly, drug-induced lupus erythematosus can occur as a side effect of some drugs, such as beta blockers, which are commonly used to treat heart disease and hypertension. Finally, neo-natal lupus erythematosus, which is a rare form of lupus in newborn babies whose mothers have lupus. It can cause problems at birth or, in rare cases, a serious heart defect.[5]

Kaleidoscope Fighting Lupus reports that an estimated figure of over five million people worldwide suffer from this debilitating disease. Of those affected with lupus, 90% are women between the ages of fifteen and forty-five, and of those, two-thirds are people of colour.[6] According to ASCIA, the Australasian Society of Clinical Immunity and Allergy, in Australia and New Zealand, lupus affects 20,000 people.[7] Whilst lupus is most common in young women, it is not unheard of in children. Most children are diagnosed during puberty (like I was). However, there are rare cases of lupus in children under the age of five. Lupus symptoms in children are very similar to adults, although they are likely to be more serious. For this reason, children are generally given more aggressive treatment that aims to control the disease before it involves the major organs.

Lupus appears to be rarer in men than women (occurring at a rate of approximately 1 man for every nine women).[8] Unlike women, who tend to develop the disease between the ages of fifteen and forty-five, there is no distinct period where men are more likely to develop lupus. Men often experience slightly different symptoms, at times more severe than in women. It seems that few people develop lupus in old age. During these years, it is generally a much milder disease.

Interestingly, lupus is far more common than well-known diseases such as leukaemia, multiple sclerosis, muscular dystrophy and cystic fibrosis combined. As of yet, lupus has no cure. Without early diagnosis and treatment, lupus can be severely debilitating, even resulting in death. However, advances in the medical and research community are continually being made, which will lead to earlier diagnosis, better treatments and hopefully a cure.

Lupus was first described back in the time of Hippocrates in Ancient Greece. The word lupus means 'wolf' in Latin. So, how was the word 'lupus' chosen? One theory is that lupus was selected because the common butterfly rash seen on the cheeks and nose of many lupus patients is similar to the facial markings of a wolf. Another theory relates to the early use of the word 'lupus' to describe skin ulcers. During the sixteenth century, certain skin ulcers were compared to a hungry wolf eating the sufferer's flesh.[9]

Whilst lupus is not a contagious disease, medical professionals and researchers cannot say for certain what causes lupus. However, it is agreed that several factors could determine a person's likelihood of developing lupus. Genetics is a possible factor. While a family history of lupus does not mean an individual will get lupus, it can determine a person's likelihood of the disease. I have read many stories where lupus runs strongly in families. The environment, which includes exposure to UV light (photosensitivity), smoking, stress or toxins, may be a contributing factor. Further research is still needed. Hormones and illness are possible factors too. Research is suggesting that higher levels of hormones such as oestrogen and progesterone are linked to autoimmune diseases such as lupus.[10] This could explain the fact that women in their childbearing years are the most common demographic afflicted with lupus. It may even explain why I developed lupus at the beginning of adolescence, a time of significant hormonal change. Medications have also been suggested as possible causes. Some medications are suspected triggers of lupus and symptom flares. This is a subset of the disease. Drug-induced lupus is based on this theory. Often, once a patient with drug-induced lupus stops taking the medications suspected of inducing lupus, the symptoms can reduce rapidly. Finally, a combination of factors could also be considered as the cause of lupus. Many in the medical and research fields believe that a person with a combination of factors such as genetics, the environment, hormones and illness or medications is likely to be more susceptible to develop lupus than a person with only one of these factors. With more funds invested into medical research, we will be one step closer to understanding the cause of lupus.

According to the Lupus Foundation of America, a variety of medicines are used to treat lupus. They range from mild to extremely strong. Prescribed medications are likely to change during a person's lifetime with lupus. However, it can take months, sometimes years, before the right combination of medicines is able to keep lupus symptoms under control. The goals of a lupus treatment plan are to control symptoms such as joint pain and fatigue, to reduce inflammation in the body, to suppress the overactive immune system, prevent flares and treat them when they occur and minimise damage to organs. The most commonly used medications for these purposes include:

- **Non-steroidal anti-inflammatory** medications such as meloxicam (Mobic®);
- **Corticosteroids** including prednisolone and prednisone;
- **Antimalarials** such as hydroxychloroquine (Plaquenil®) and chloroquine;
- **Immunosuppressants** such as azathioprine (Imuran®), methotrexate (Rheumatrex™) and cyclophosphamide (Cytoxan®);
- **Biologics** such as the monoclonal antibody belimumab (Benlysta®). This is the first drug to be specifically developed for lupus in over sixty years;
- **Anticoagulants** such as aspirin, heparin (Calciparine®) and warfarin (Coumadin®).[11]

So, What Is Lupus?

* * *

At the time of writing this book, I am currently taking the NSAID (which stands for non-steroidal anti-inflammatory drug) Mobic, the antimalarial hydroxychloroquine, the immunosuppressant methotrexate and a complementary medicine called DHEA (dehydroepiandrosterone), an endogenous steroid used as an additional energy source to combat fatigue. I also take short rounds of the corticosteroid prednisolone when I am having a lupus flare. The doses of these medications are modified at times due to the state of my lupus. For example, sometimes I need to take a higher dose of methotrexate if I am having concurrent lupus flares. The aim here is to reduce inflammation and possible organ damage. When my lupus appears to be more controlled, the dose of methotrexate is likely to be reduced again. The desired treatment plan is to be on the lowest doses as possible of these medications.

After nearly twenty years of chronic corticosteroid use, I was advised by my current rheumatologist to stop. Corticosteroids can cause damage to the density of the bones, including the development of conditions such as osteoporosis and various other long-term side effects. I had developed the bone condition osteopenia as a result of chronic, long-term corticosteroid use. The ageing process, as well as being female, were also seen as risk factors for further reduced bone density and increased likelihood of bone fractures. My chronic corticosteroid use was already a significant risk factor, so it was decided that trialling life without corticosteroids was my best option of reducing the likelihood of further bone density issues as I age.

Tapering off corticosteroids was a long process. It took me over a year to completely ween off them. This was a challenging time, as my body was so used to having this medication every day for nearly twenty years. Of all my medications, this was the one that gave me the energy I needed to complete regular activities each day. It gave me wings! I needed to take time off work for this process to be successful, which thankfully it was, but I do feel more fatigued without it. I now only take short doses of corticosteroids when my lupus is flaring, in conjunction with a myriad of other immune suppressants. This way, I am treating the disease when it is extremely active, without subjecting my body to further damage due to prolonged, chronic corticosteroid use.

Being immunosuppressed is fraught with the possibility of many nasty side effects. Lupus Warriors have additional worries when taking these medications. I try to remember that these drugs are keeping me alive and giving me the quality of life I am now able to have. And that is a blessing.

Once diagnosed with lupus, you are likely to be referred to see a rheumatologist for ongoing treatment. A rheumatologist is a doctor who specialises in diseases of the joints and muscles. They are likely to work closely with you to develop a wellness and treatment plan that takes into consideration your age, symptoms and lifestyle. The aim in managing lupus symptoms is to reduce inflammation in the body caused by lupus and suppress the overactive immune system, prevent flares and treat them as soon as they occur, control symptoms such as joint pain and fatigue, and minimise damage to organs in the body.

If lupus has caused damage to a particular organ, other specialists are consulted. For example, a cardiologist for heart disease, a dermatologist for cutaneous lupus, a nephrologist for kidney disease, a neurologist for brain and nervous system disease or a gastroenterologist for gastrointestinal disease, just to name a few.

What can be expected when living with lupus? Lupus is different for each individual, but it often appears in cycles, which can consist of:

- a 'flare', with severe acute symptoms needing medical attention;
- a 'chronic' phase, when symptoms may continue but are less severe; and
- a 'remission', when symptoms may disappear completely for long periods of time but can still return.[12]

* * *

During the chronic phase, and especially in the remission phase, a person with lupus needs to avoid situations that can possibly cause a flare. These include becoming too tired, stressed, poor diet or other factors that are likely to be noticed by the patient or their doctors. My lupus has never gone into a period of remission.

What is the prognosis for lupus patients? Pleasingly, the prognosis of lupus is better today than ever before. With regular follow-up and treatment, 80-90% of people with lupus can expect to live a normal lifespan. As medical science is yet to develop a cure for lupus, people do die from this disease. However, for the majority of people diagnosed with lupus, it will not be fatal.[13]

Lupus varies in intensity and degree. Some people have a mild case, others moderate and some severe, which is likely to be more difficult to treat and control. For people who have a severe flare-up, there is a greater chance that their lupus may be life threatening. People with non-organ threatening symptoms of lupus can look forward to a normal lifespan if they follow the instructions of their physicians, take their medications regularly as prescribed and know when to seek help when experiencing unexpected side-effects of a medication or the manifestation of new lupus symptoms.

Although some people with lupus have severe recurrent attacks that result in hospitalisation, most rarely require hospitalisation. In particular, hospital visits are rare for those lupus patients who maintain a healthy lifestyle and are vigilant in their care of managing lupus symptoms.

For people suffering from an autoimmune disease such as lupus, unfortunately, they are also at risk of developing more than one autoimmune disease.[14] Sjogren's syndrome is commonly experienced by lupus sufferers. It is an autoimmune disease that attacks glands in the lining in and around the eyes, mouth and genitals. These linings usually secrete fluid to keep these areas moist. In Sjogren's syndrome, the eyes, mouth and often genitals, become extremely dry, as the secretion of moisture in these linings is significantly reduced. Eye drops, creams and fluids, amongst many other products, can help to restore lost moisture and ease discomfort induced from these symptoms. Thyroid disease, coeliac disease and Raynaud's phenomenon are also common conditions developed by those with lupus. I suffer from both Sjogren's syndrome and Raynaud's phenomenon, as well as a suspected thyroid disease.

* * *

Whilst lupus is a serious disease, diagnosis and treatment are improving. The progress made in these areas during the last decade has been greater than that made over the past 100 years. Hopefully, more advancements in lupus education and awareness can continue to evolve, particularly in the earlier diagnosis of the disease, which is critical in helping to prevent the development of life-threatening organ damage.

Whilst it took three long years for my own lupus diagnosis, in many ways I am fortunate, for at this stage of my life, I have showed no signs of organ damage. I attribute this to my young age when diagnosed and effective intervention of immunosuppressants, which helped to control my lupus symptoms. Hopefully, this has been significant in reducing the prospect of organ damage for me in the future. So many lupus patients, particularly women in their child-bearing years, appear to have endured undiagnosed, untreated lupus symptoms for many years that have resulted in severe, life-threatening organ damage. Lupus symptoms such as extreme fatigue, headaches, fever and achy muscles and joints, can be easily dismissed by women as being attributed to motherhood or work-related stress, resulting in prolonged diagnosis and treatment, and hence, causing more severe, life-threatening forms of this insidious disease.

Worse yet, so many doctors in the medical profession don't consider lupus as a possible cause of these symptoms. While they are likely to know its name and have a vague understanding of some of its symptoms, I know personally to this day the ignorance of some GPs, in particular, when it comes to lupus. Did they miss the lecture on lupus during their medical training? I have lost count as to how many times I have had to explain symptoms and medications needed to treat lupus during a doctor's consultation. After having lupus for thirty years, I find the general understanding of lupus in the medical world frustrating and ultimately frightening. We need more support, for without more education and awareness of lupus and its devasting effects, how will we ever find a cure?

Part Two

Persevere

Adjusting to My New Normal

Chapter Nine

So, I Have Lupus

'Hey, Rachel! How come your face is so fat but the rest of your body is normal?' Another comment about my weight. My somewhat 'bloated' appearance. They kept coming.

'Rachel? You're not Rachel. You don't look anything like her at all.' Extremely embarrassed and humiliated in front of other students, I presented my concession card as a form of ID to my former Year 8 Greek teacher, who refused to believe that I was the Rachel Lea she had taught only a few years before.

I could cope with people's interest. I could cope with people's concern. But what I couldn't cope with was the physical changes that were happening to me, for all to see, or the barrage of insensitive comments that people felt compelled to share. Why did everyone have to make a comment about my changed appearance? Didn't they know how shy I was, how difficult it was to be given extra attention in this way? Why couldn't they be happy that I was getting well, feeling better and attending full days at school? Why, oh why, hadn't anyone heard of lupus?

As a result of my high, daily dose of corticosteroids, I had developed Cushing's syndrome. Cushing's syndrome is a disorder that occurs when the body is exposed to high levels of the hormone cortisol for a long time. It is likely to be caused by the use of oral corticosteroid medications. Our body naturally makes cortisol, but I was having an extra amount on top of what my body was making in the form of these corticosteroids. Symptoms of Cushing's syndrome include weight gain and fatty tissue deposits, particularly around the face (known as 'moon face'), the lower abdomen and upper back, creating what's known as a 'buffalo hump'.[15] I developed weight gain, mainly in the face and lower abdomen, making me look extremely bloated. My face felt sore and swollen, and it became difficult to smile and eat as it was painful to move the muscles in my face.

My bloated face was quite visible but thankfully I was able to conceal most of the other physical changes that were occurring, such as dramatic changes in my skin. My body was gaining weight at such a dramatic rate, the strain of such intense physical growth was causing stretch marks. Within a week of taking the corticosteroids, the Cushing's syndrome had created large, purple and reddish stretch marks all over my legs known as striae. These could not be concealed when wearing my summer school dress. Thankfully, they appeared on the inside of my legs and upper thigh area, so anyone who did notice would have had to be staring at my legs for way too long and very inappropriately! To this day, I have scars on my legs from these stretch marks. They have never fully healed, probably because I have been on chronic immunosuppressant medication for thirty years, which reduces the body's ability to heal.

In addition to these stretch marks, I started to bruise very easily. Knocking into the corners of tables or doorways and the like, I became sensitive to being bruised. Huge purple bruises appeared and took a while to heal. My skin was becoming thinner, due to Cushing's syndrome, which contributed to these bruises. My muscles were also becoming weaker. They were already deconditioned due to being sedentary and inactive for so long. It was quite frustrating trying to feel strong enough to exercise more. Losing the strength in my muscles made it even more difficult to find a way to build them back up without overexerting myself.

Taking prolonged, high doses of corticosteroids meant that my bones were also at risk of becoming thinner and of developing the bone condition known as osteoporosis. Whilst taking this medication, I needed to begin regular bone scans to monitor their strength and to see if they were becoming porous and susceptible to fractures. It became another worry during this time, as I was taking corticosteroids indefinitely and the likelihood of developing osteoporosis was very high.

My mood also began to change. Always a quiet, gentle, cooperative girl, I began a roller coaster of emotions each day. In one day, I could swing from feeling bright, energetic, even euphoric, to feeling very teary and depressed, even angry and aggressive. Being able to control my emotions was challenging. The steroids were in control of how I was feeling now. I just had to ride each wave, each day, the best way I could. I had to remind myself that if I was feeling a little differently from my usual self, this was the steroid's doing, not mine.

Another significant change was my appetite. I became increasingly hungry most of the time. A main meal would not sustain me. My stomach would begin growling an hour or so later; hollow and empty and demanding to be refilled. It was a very annoying feeling, knowing that I had eaten enough but that my body was yearning for more. I had to learn to drink more fluids and not over-snack to avoid gaining even more weight than all of the fluid that my body had begun to accumulate. Aside from my bloated face, I developed a hunched upper back and more fluid in this area as well. The back of my knees produced sacks of fluid too – very unsightly for a teenager! Another significant change was more bloating in my lower abdomen. I looked four months pregnant – I'm not kidding. I felt heavy in this area and was constantly peeing in the loo. This meant waking up in the night too often, which would impact on the quality of sleep I would get.

I was also sweating profusely, as if I had been running a marathon. It was extremely embarrassing and affected the colour choice of clothing I wore. I did everything I could to cover up any unsightly sweaty marks. Dark-coloured tops were out as they would clearly highlight my sweating problem. Acne on my face also appeared more severely, another visual reminder of what this medication was doing to me physically. Adolescence was hard enough without the added anxiety of illness and side-effects from toxic medication. Though frustrating, it quickly humbled me. I had no right to complain. Why? Well simply, this drug was saving my life.

Aside from these changes, the biggest challenge I experienced was my increased risk of contracting infections. As corticosteroids were supressing and shutting down my body's immune system, I was susceptible to catching infections very easily. This predisposition to infection made attending school regularly very difficult. It was such an irony as here I was, finally able to take some medication to ease my pain and fatigue, boosting my energy and helping me to feel strong enough to attend school. On the flip side, I was catching every cold that was going around at school. An average cold was not just so for me. When I would catch a cold, it would linger for weeks and took ages to truly break. For example, instead of having a sore throat for a couple of days, then the blocked, runny rose and then the cough, I would have the sore throat for a week or more as the infection tried to figure out what to do next. My supressed immune system didn't quite know what to do when foreign agents appeared, as it was busy fighting my own cells, which it incorrectly recognised as enemy cells. Sometimes I would be out of school for a week or two trying to overcome a cold. It became very draining, not to mention frustrating, as I would fall further behind with my homework.

In addition to this, I was also having chronic urinary tract infections and chronic vaginal thrush. My parents were frequently taking me to the GP's to get prescriptions for more medicines, and then off to the chemist, paying for expensive creams to help treat these infections. The infections would then clear up but, within a week or two, they would return and off to the GP we would go again. I felt so much for my parents. As I have said previously, we were a family of five on one income, and I felt so bad that the chronic infections I was contracting were so costly to treat. The frequent specialist appointments, purchase of corticosteroids and anti-inflammatories were costly enough. Steroids were extremely expensive in the nineties. The addition of purchasing antibiotics and creams made it even more challenging for them. My parents never made me feel guilty or spoke a word to me about these additional expenses, but I knew that they were battling with this financial hardship. Stoic as always, they persevered with much grace and humility. It was inspiring for me to see how dignified they were at this time (and still are to this day), and how to truly rise up to life's many challenges.

In saying this, with much humility, I should extend this compliment to myself. Looking back now, I am amazed by how well I coped during this time. There I was, newly diagnosed with an incurable disease, returning to school after a significant absence and then having to battle the effects of steroids and these pesky infections all the time; it was a lot for a young woman of sixteen years old to adjust to. However, I truly don't recall being a difficult teenager or going through the classic teenage years of brooding or being demanding. I was never slamming doors or screaming at my parents for not understanding me or isolating myself from the world, cooped up in my bedroom in an adolescent funk. In retrospect, I don't think anyone in my family would have been too upset with me if I did become a little antsy or lashed out in a state of self-pity. Mum, Dad, Ross and Rebecca had a front row seat to my ongoing anguish. They saw how much lupus was changing my regular life. Remarkably, it was for the better. Knowingly or unknowingly, I was learning and developing greater insight and an appreciation for how lucky I was.

Whilst I did have my moments of tears and breaking down in frustration from feeling chronically unwell and at the mercy of these steroids, it was always temporary and replaced by my resolve to keep looking forward and to be grateful for what I was well enough to be able to do. At this age, I somehow knew that I needed a positive approach to life to enable me to fight this disease. I only had to think of how long I had spent in my bed or how difficult it used to be to walk and I could quickly find perspective and solace in how far I had come. It was really that simple.

The negative side-effects of taking steroids were quite extensive and challenging, but I owed them much gratitude for helping me to be a functional person again. Steroids induced and awakened a spiritedness within me that I had not felt in years. I was smiling as widely as I could, laughing loud and long and feeling so much more strength in every step I took. The energy that I now had surged through me. The happiness I now exuded was a gift. It was truly wonderful. Not to mention the fact that I now had a major medication to help my body fight this disease called lupus.

Although it did take a long time to diagnose, any longer without the aid of these steroids I most likely would have suffered more acutely from organ damage due to lupus. I felt so grateful that I was able to receive a diagnosis when I did because beginning this new steroid treatment helped to stop this disease from doing even more damage than it had already done. At that time, I didn't want to imagine what life could have looked like for me if I remained undiagnosed and untreated. Well, it didn't bare thinking about.

It was also the relief I felt by now knowing what I had been suffering from all this time was still deep within me. The relief of knowing that I was not making up the severity of my symptoms and the pain I was in was profound. It had been quite debilitating being dismissed by many of the medical practitioners we had met as not being in pain or that what I was feeling was temporary and nothing to worry about. I had suppressed much anger at being made to doubt myself for all of those years. To be a young, teenage girl and not be taken seriously really did clip my wings and break my spirit.

So, it truly was an immediate acceptance the minute it was confirmed that I had lupus. I embraced the name and the medication that I could now take. It was as if the missing pieces to a jigsaw puzzle had been found and popped back into place with ease and clarity, for I could now make plans for my future. I could look ahead and start dreaming with more hope in my heart – that I was, hopefully, going to be okay.

Chapter Ten

VCE On Steroids

Aside from adjusting to this new diagnosis, the impact of steroids and battling chronic infections, I had the task of reconnecting with school life. As I had been diagnosed with lupus and begun steroid treatment at the end of the summer holidays, it was very timely in helping me in my transition back to school. I was feeling very hopeful that I would be strong enough to attend school on a regular basis. The pain in my joints and muscles continued to improve. I was less fatigued and the energy the steroids were giving me was a gift. I would still have a little nap each day but I didn't fall asleep anymore. What a difference!

However, my life as a Year 11 VCE student was spent very much on the periphery. Even though I had attended school intermittently at the end of the previous year, I still found being back at school very overwhelming to begin with. I was fortunate to have friends and people I knew in each of my classes, but these friendships were not close ones. My friends shared stories of their lives that seemed completely foreign to mine. Stories of boyfriends and going out at night, even sneaking into nightclubs in the city. Of parties and new clothes and part-time jobs. Stories of freedom and independence. All were told with ease and normality (and no doubt, much bravado). No one shared stories of doctors and hospital visits, medications taken or how sick they felt. No one spoke of their fear for remaining well and in good health so that they could complete their VCE and get into uni. No one shared stories of being diagnosed with an incurable, potentially fatal disease.

I was very much on the outside looking in and a huge part of me felt in awe of how easy everyone's lives appeared. Effortless. No worries. I would be lying if I said that I didn't feel slightly envious. I had no one to really share my experiences with. I was free from the daily confines of my bedroom but I was still isolated. I tried very hard not to feel too lonely about it, even though I was. Thankfully, the demands of school and managing my lupus kept me busy enough so that I didn't languish too long in feeling sorry for myself.

During a moment of peer pressure at school one day, I unwillingly accepted an invitation to a sixteenth birthday party for a girl in one of my classes. I wasn't overly friendly with her and was bemused by my invitation in the first place. She was a loud, talkative girl and I didn't have much in common with her. I was very anxious about going to this party, but my parents agreed that even though I was not a close friend of this girl, it would be a good opportunity to mix with other kids outside of the classroom. I agonised over what to wear – all of the typical neuroses this age brings. It was a big deal for me as I had missed so many of these opportunities to socialise when I was ill.

When I arrived at this party, I felt even more out of place than I did at school. I hardly knew anyone there. And it was boring. So boring! I wanted to go home not long after arriving. When it was time to go, I felt so relieved. I had spent the entire night standing around watching other kids my age basically talk crap and behave in a way that I could not relate to. They were obsessed with talking about alcohol or having a sneaky cigarette. I was not interested in drinking alcohol or getting off my face or smoking or doing anything that, socially, I was meant to be experimenting with at this age. I was already a mature young person before lupus came along. But having lupus was an absolute game changer in every area of my life.

Being at this party brought it home to me that I was not like everyone else my age. My worries were deeply embedded in how I managed to get through each day. Whilst my peers were stressing about picking up boys or how to get alcohol, I was worried for my life and what would become of me. How could I be expected to relate? I was processing and adapting to the diagnosis of a life-long, incurable disease. My prognosis was unclear. There was a question mark hanging over everything I did. Will I make it through a day at school? Will I be well enough to walk home from school each day? Will I finish the term? Will I pass Year 11? What will my future look like? Will I live a long life? No wonder I felt so alone.

I also felt very self-conscious in regard to my learning capabilities. I had missed so much school and it was a loss I felt deeply. My classmates seemed more confident and assured than me. I was completing the bare minimum of subjects, 4 per unit for my VCE, each semester. I felt very aware of the limited subject choices I had been given. Although my record as an outstanding student had influenced the school's decision to allow me to continue at Year 11, it made me feel a little sad that I was unable to pick any subject I wanted to, like everyone else. I had to select subjects that reflected my absences. I had to be realistic and not select subjects that were beyond my abilities or that would be too stressful to complete due to missing out on so much prior content.

Science subjects such as Biology, Chemistry or Physics were too content-heavy and complex to even consider. Physical Education was out of the question for obvious reasons. I was in no condition at that time to be running laps at school! English was a compulsory subject so one out of four subjects was already decided for me. At that time, somewhere within my sixteen units of VCE subjects, I had to complete two units of a Mathematics class to satisfactorily pass my VCE. As I had missed Year 10 Mathematics, I had no choice but to select the bottom level class called Space and Numbers. In teenage speak, this was translated as 'Veggie Maths'. It was for all of the students who struggled with maths. As maths was not my strong point or my favourite, it didn't worry me too much. I knew that there was no way I would cope with any of the other math classes that were more demanding and for super math wizzes. So that left only two choices left. I loved reading books, so selecting Literature was thankfully an easy choice. I hoped I could bounce back quickly in this subject.

The last subject selected was Health Education. I felt drawn to this subject given my health battles, and I was interested to see what we would learn. Overall, I was hopeful that I could pass these subjects if I did my best. I was also awarded more spare periods within my daily timetable because I was not completing the required VCE units like everyone else.

This was a reassuring outcome, as I could sit in the library and work at my own pace on my homework (or even better, I could just sit, rest and relax a little!)

After a few months of taking a high steroid dosage at the beginning of Year 11, my doctors at the Royal Children's Hospital felt that it was time to reduce the dose. The goal at the beginning of the steroid regime was to hit the disease hard, and once improvement in my symptoms could be seen, the dose would then be reduced. Thankfully, my symptoms were improving and my doctors were encouraged by my progress and the likelihood that I could function on a reduced steroid dose on a daily basis. The rheumatologist devised a plan for me to taper off the steroids. I had taken 75mg for two weeks, then 50mg for the next three weeks. I was to then take 50mg on each alternate day, dropping by 5mg each week until 25mg on alternate days was reached. I was then to ring my rheumatologist and report my progress. The next step was to then keep tapering the dosage down each week by 5mg until I reached 5mg, taking this each alternate day indefinitely.

This tapering plan literally never went to plan. New to the regime of tapering off corticosteroids, I was unaware of the nightmare experience I was about to endure. A few days before I was due to start tapering, I had been battling a bladder infection. Once that cleared, it was straight into the steroid plan. There was not much reprieve. The day came for skipping the regular 50mg steroid dose. I always took my steroids straight after breakfast and at the same time each morning. It was important for my body to have a regular routine when taking steroids. I had learned early on that if I was slightly late in taking it, I would start to feel agitated and unwell.

The morning appeared to begin well but before too long, I started to experience severe withdrawal symptoms. I started to experience intense stabbing and aching pains throughout my knees and legs. It felt as though someone was stabbing me with a knife. I could hardly keep my eyes open. I was writhing on the couch in pain and quite distressed. I was in this state for about twelve hours straight. At this point, I had gone without steroids for approximately thirty-seven hours. My parents and I assumed that what I was experiencing was normal when tapering off the steroids, so they monitored me and I endured this discomfort the best way I could.

I took the scheduled dose of steroids the following day. It took a couple of hours, but the stabbing pains started to ease. I felt a little relief but my muscles felt very tender, possibly due to all of that pain. Unfortunately, these stabbing pains returned later in the day. Mum was frantic. It had been distressing for her to see me suffering like this. I was quite terrified. Taking this medication was a whole new experience for me, and for my parents. We were so confused. We had executed every single step of the rheumatologist's steroid tapering plan. Why was this happening? Was this the normal reaction? We didn't think so, as the rheumatologist had assured my parents and I that I would not experience any withdrawal symptoms.

Mum was able to reach my paediatrician at the Royal Children's Hospital by phone. My paediatrician was in disbelief when learning of the withdrawal experience I had endured. She told Mum that what I experienced shouldn't have happened. This normally calm, pleasant lady became quite defensive and uncompromising. Mum was furious, because it did happen and I had suffered a severe, serious reaction. My paediatrician didn't appear to be concerned by the withdrawal side effects I had experienced and was in full support of my rheumatologist's actions.

She instructed Mum to continue administering the original steroid tapering plan. Mum was still extremely concerned that the response I was having was not normal, so she rang the now former Victorian Lupus Association for further advice. The person Mum spoke to was extremely supportive and worried that my response was not normal and recommended that Mum take me to the emergency department at the Austin Hospital for monitoring.

My parents bundled me into the car and took me straight to the emergency department at the Austin Hospital. When I was eventually seen to, I was examined by a female GP for what seemed like forever. She was concerned that not taking 50mg, a high steroid dose, every alternate day, was too much for my young body to withstand. I was at risk of having a heart attack due to the stress and craving my body was experiencing, yearning for the next steroid intake. She was quite perplexed that I was expected to go one day without taking steroids of such a high dose. Steroids are an incredibly addictive medication and my body was demanding the next dose.

Concerned about the next best course of action, this doctor was able to contact my rheumatologist for advice. My rheumatologist demanded to speak to Mum on the phone, instead of the GP. Mum was so angry at what was happening to me, she refused to speak to him. The GP tried very hard to change Mum's mind but she absolutely refused. So, my rheumatologist spoke at length to the GP, devising an alternate steroid tapering plan that would hopefully not be so painful.

I stayed in the emergency ward for a little while as my heart rate was monitored. I was quite agitated and my pulse was racing. When I had stabilised, I was sent home. The steroids began to kick in and I started to feel better. But I was very exhausted by the whole process and needed to take it easy for a few days until my body re-adjusted to regularly taking steroids each day again.

Frustrated and concerned that the rheumatologist and paediatrician were not experienced enough in treating a young woman with lupus, my parents sought a referral from my GP for me to see an experienced adult rheumatologist, who had been recommended by a supportive person from the Victorian Lupus Association. I was in that difficult category – half child, half adult – as a sixteen-year-old girl. My parents were concerned that the original steroid tapering plan was not suitable for someone my age. This meant that I would no longer be in the care of the rheumatologist or paediatrician at the Royal Children's Hospital. My parents wrote to both doctors and thanked them for all they had done for me. They organised for my records to be transferred to my new rheumatologist.

I had to wait a few months to see the new rheumatologist. I was able to continue tapering my steroids, very slowly, according to the revised plan. When the first appointment came around, it was another anxious moment of having to be scrutinised by another doctor. This one was a male, aged in his late forties. My first impressions found him to be polite, thorough and extremely knowledgeable about lupus, but he was quite brisk and slightly arrogant – very definitive about the course of action my treatment would be.

He was grateful for the medical history compiled by my parents. It had been such an arduous process in diagnosing my lupus, let alone to explain it verbally, so it was helpful for him to read my timeline of symptoms and assess how they had manifested. He too, was concerned about the original steroid tapering plan, agreeing that it was dangerous to go without a high dose of steroids for a whole day. He restructured my steroid tapering plan so that reducing my dose was more manageable. At the end of the consultation, the rheumatologist agreed to see me regularly as a permanent patient.

My parents and I left his office that day feeling hopeful about the medical care I would now be receiving. According to my GP, this rheumatologist was extremely revered by his peers and I would be in good hands. It was a relief to know that I would be seeing a doctor who specialised in treating lupus patients and that his experience would be of benefit to my health and well-being.

The remainder of Year 11 was the continued journey of adapting to steroids, managing my fatigue and pain and to fighting back from chronic infections. Colds and bladder infections such as cystitis and Candida infections continued to dominate my life. Steroids had reduced my immunity as they are an immunosuppressant medication. I continued to be very conscious of being around people with colds and infections as I was a sitting duck for catching them.

I managed my schoolwork the best way I could. My teachers were very supportive. If I was unable to meet a deadline, extensions were provided for me. This was so helpful in reducing the stress associated with being a VCE student. Having more spare periods during the school day was also a blessing. I always needed extra time to complete my work. I was still finding it very difficult to write. I still wore my tubey foam on my fingers but, thankfully, the severity of chilblains had reduced, making it slightly less painful to write. As my intake of steroids progressed throughout the year, I noticed the pain and mobility of my fingers slightly improved too. I was able to stretch my fingers with a little more strength.

To help me complete my schoolwork, my parents bought me an electronic typewriter. It was the kind of typewriter where prior to hitting the enter key, you had to write a full line first. When you hit the enter key, it would print that line directly onto the page. It was a little stressful to begin with, as I had to make sure I had not made a mistake! Thankfully, there was a screen that you could read and check your work before you hit enter. It was amazing to be able to finally move my fingers more freely on the keyboard, compared with the distressing experience I had in Year 9 as a keyboard student in that awful Information Technology class. Steroids were reducing the inflammation in my hands, resulting in less pain and enabling more flexibility and movement in my fingers. My confidence bloomed in my ability to find the keys with much more ease. I was so grateful to have another tool to help me complete my work, as holding a pen or pencil still proved to be painful after a period of time.

My acceptance of being a lupus sufferer was ongoing. My friends at school didn't mention it so neither did I. I just longed to blend in and not be singled out with any extra attention, which is why I found it very confronting to share my experience as a lupus sufferer in my Health Education class. Our assignment was to research a disease that we didn't know much about. My lovely Health Education teacher, Mrs Jayne Walsh, suggested that I research lupus. She thought it would be helpful for me to know more about what I was suffering from and a good opportunity for the class to learn more about this little-known disease. So, I followed her advice and compiled my report on lupus. At the time, the Victorian Lupus Association was in operation and they were extremely helpful in sending me some information.

Once we had completed our reports, we had to then compile a fact sheet for the class on our chosen disease and present our report to the class. As you can imagine, I found this very confronting. I was anxious about the emotion that talking about lupus would likely bring, but I was more worked up about speaking in front of the class. I was still such a shy girl and the thought of everyone in class staring at me as I shared my private suffering was an overwhelming thought.

Amazingly, I got through it and students were really complimentary and supportive of my talk. Looking back, I can see why my Health Education teacher wanted me to talk about lupus in front of others. She knew how shy I was but wanted to help bring me out of my shell. She could see the importance of normalising my suffering and the positive impact that would bring to my life at school. She was right. I couldn't hide from being a sick student at school. Everyone knew I was sick and that I was different, but I had to become more comfortable speaking about being sick, which meant that I had to become more at ease talking about myself. I knew in my heart that I wasn't ashamed of having lupus. I had accepted that I was sick and had accepted that this sickness was called lupus. I knew it wasn't my fault that I was sick. Having lupus could happen to anyone. Anyone just happened to be me.

What I struggled with was having to disclose a personal part of myself to others, that made my life different from everyone at school. I resented this very much because lupus had interrupted my wish to be a quiet, no-fuss, completely under-the-radar student. I was mastering that life quite well before lupus came along. I did not wish to stand out in any way. But lupus had the upper hand, every time. And as an incurable disease, it was going to continue to do so – every single time.

Chapter Eleven

Discovering Strength in Perseverance

It was truly remarkable. I was sleeping well, awaking with more energy and less pain. I was so overjoyed by the improvements I was making due to being on steroids. The other medications were doing their bit, I was sure, but the impact of steroids was so powerful, so visceral. I could feel them flowing through me. My body would let me know if I was late in taking them. I would become weary and agitated very quickly, ready for my next fix. I was clearly addicted. My body had changed from being an extremely healthy, rarely medicated being, to a disease-ridden, steroid and pain killer pumping figure.

My young body had experienced so many changes. It had been invaded by a disease that changed its cellular make-up so severely, that it didn't recognise its own cells anymore. I had become my own worst enemy – literally. Effectively at war with itself every minute, every second, of every day. My body was trying to attack itself and destroy all of the growth and development it had achieved since I had been conceived. The introduction of toxic chemicals in the form of all of these medications was no doubt an unfamiliar and resentful presence. My regular bodily functions had been interrupted by these foreign agents. Much adjustment was needed to embrace them for the goodness they were trying to bring, for they were the army that was built to turn my cells around and bring peace to this ongoing war in my body.

I didn't have time to be a moody, sullen or ungrateful teenager. I had skipped that station. I was fast-tracked to a place where having perspective and wisdom were needed if I was to join this army of chemical warfare and be at peace with the uncontrollable changes that had happened to me. If my attitude was not positive, hopeful or realistic, I would be harming all of the good work this army was trying to achieve. I embraced this responsibility because I was lucky. I was lucky because I loved and cared about myself. I was lucky because for the first time since I had become unwell, I was able to take medication that was trying to save my life. I didn't want to let my army down. And so, my new life as a Lupus Warrior had truly begun.

***

I marched into Year 12 feeling victorious. I had passed Year 11. It was an amazing feeling to know that in being given a chance to complete my VCE within the constraints of limited subject choices, I had managed to satisfactorily meet all of the expectations that my fellow students were also meeting. It mattered so much to me to be able to keep up and reach the same academic milestones as my peers.

Because of these achievements, I approached Year 12 with much hope. My subject selection was different from Year 11. I still had to complete English but I was unable to continue studying Literature or Health Education due to poor student interest. There simply was not enough students to warrant running classes for these two subjects, which was a real shame. However, an exciting new subject called Psychology was being introduced into the VCE curriculum for the first time. As my subject choices were very limited, I selected this subject because I would be on the same page as everyone else; we would all be completing this subject for the first time together. That left two more subjects to choose. A subject called Human Development piqued my interest. It focused on human growth and development throughout the lifespan and incorporated the study of many nutritional topics that were of interest to me.

My final choice, surprisingly, was PE (Physical Education). Whilst I had not anticipated that this subject would be a part of my allotment, on closer examination, it fitted in really well with Human Development and Psychology. All three subjects were connected in their examination of the human body. Whilst there was a small component of compulsory physical activity in completing PE, these requirements could be modified to meet my physical capabilities. If I was well enough to participate, great. If not, that was fine too. The majority of the subject was heavily theory based, which I was relieved about. I felt really happy about studying all four of these subjects. I just had to maintain my health. And pass! For I was so close but so far away from completing my VCE; a truly momentous milestone considering all of the challenges I was experiencing.

I continued having support from the District Teachers Association. My visiting teacher, Jackie, continued liaising with my teachers at school. She organised regular student support group meetings throughout the year with myself, my teachers and my parents. We continued to discuss the progress I was making and the special considerations that needed to be put into effect in order for me to complete work requirements. I felt very comforted by the care I was being given. It helped to ease my worries.

One of the most worrying issues for me was the completion of external end-of-year exams. I was very anxious about being able to complete my exams within the designated time period. Even though I was now taking steroids and other medications that were increasing the mobility in my hands, it still took me a long time to write. Holding a pencil felt softer than the harsh plastic of a pen. Thankfully, with much investigation from the VCE coordinator and my visiting teacher, I was awarded more time to complete my exams. I felt very relieved about this. When the time for my exams came, I needed that extra time very much.

I was also awarded extended time to complete the myriad of Work Requirements and Common Assessment Tasks, known as CATs, if I needed it. CATs were huge tasks that were completed over many months. They were predominantly research tasks that required many drafts that were corrected by our teachers. As students, we would then amend our work, submit another draft for marking and so on until it was near perfect to submit as the completed CAT by the due date. It was so reassuring to know that if I was ill and fell behind schedule, I had that extra time to complete my work to the best of my ability.

It was not lost on me that I was very fortunate to have support in place if and when I needed it. It was also remarkable to learn that the school had never implemented special considerations like mine for other VCE students before. VCE was very new at that time, having crossed over from the previous HSC (High School Certificate) system in Victoria. It was hard to comprehend that there hadn't been medical issues with previous students that would have paved the way for me in regard to the organisation of my special needs. Without fully comprehending it at the time, my illness was teaching my teachers how to re-examine their approach to delivering a truly holistic and inclusive curriculum. They were learning how to modify existing administrative procedures and how to facilitate my needs within the context of Department of Education standards. They were being challenged too. And it was a most positive series of professional challenges for them, for it would encourage greater awareness of students suffering from chronic illnesses and knowing how to address their special needs in completing their VCE in the future.

* * *

I approached the demands of completing my Year 12 studies with the same determination and focus that I had given my Year 11 subjects. The fear of failure was very present in my conscious, and it mattered so much that I gave my absolute best to each and every one of my subjects. I didn't want to waste the opportunities I was receiving. My brother, sister and I were raised to always be grateful, to be appreciative of what we had and not get caught up in comparing ourselves with others and what we didn't have.

In being well enough to participate in the completion of my secondary education, I was full of gratitude, but it was challenging to be around so many of my friends and peers who were, simply, directionless. They drifted through their studies without any awareness of how lucky they were to be healthy and well. If they failed a subject, they had enough in their VCE subject load to pass satisfactorily. They were well enough to have part-time jobs and boyfriends. Well enough to have money and energy to go out most weekends. They were able to save, get their licenses and buy cars. When they spoke, everything sounded so easy. There was such certainty in how they spoke. Conversations were prefaced with, 'when I get my licence' or 'when I get into uni.' There were no 'ifs' or 'maybes'. Everything was simply, a matter of when. It was quite foolish to me that my friends could dare to speak so assuredly and with so much confidence. It was as if they had complete control over their lives. That life was going to bring them what they wanted, when they wanted it. I just couldn't relate.

Lupus was not only isolating me physically but socially and mentally as well. I would feel quite flat at times just listening to what they were able to do – so many things that I wasn't well enough to do. It was hard. I had to rest after school and on weekends and pace myself if I had any chance of completing Year 12 successfully. The worries I had were always churning away internally. All I could do was to keep following the advice of my parents, which was to focus on what I was able to do and just do my very best. It was not going to be helpful, no matter how envious I was at the ease of other people's lives, to compare myself with everyone around me, for I was still standing with strength and determination, despite the uncertainty ahead. I was trying to make every day count and that hopefully I would be able to complete the end of my final year of secondary school, knowing I had cherished every step.

Having this perspective was integral in maintaining a positive attitude. But I wasn't always successful in putting this perspective into practice. Yes, a lupus diagnosis had been made but that was just the beginning. The journey to acceptance of this disease and its intrusion into my life was my next challenge. Mature as I was, I was still a teenager, not to mention one with steroids coursing through her veins! I had moments when I was very defiant in the face of the limitations that lupus was enforcing on me.

PE class was probably the subject where my limitations were flashing loudly in my face. Every few weeks, we would have a class that focused on physical activity, such as basketball, rock climbing, snooker – a wide range of fun, tactile activities that required physical activity and participation from everyone in the class. Whilst I had been given much support by my PE teacher that I wasn't expected to participate if I didn't feel up to it, on many occasions I ignored this advice. I was determined to join in with everyone else and not be the girl sitting on the sidelines. I had spent so much of my schooling sitting on the outer that my yearning to be just like everyone else took over any common sense I had and I would do things that I probably shouldn't have.

I remember the week we focused on basketball. The class was split into two teams. I had assured my teacher that I was strong enough to join in and play. I must have been feeling super energetic that day because I had never played a game of basketball in my life, but I managed to run, be agile and quick on my feet and even pass and shoot the ball with such power that I nearly knocked out one of the boys by throwing the ball at his head unintentionally! I surprised myself. And it was both scary and exciting. It felt so good to be a part of the team and in that moment to just throw that ball and feel carefree. I had so much fun, which was the biggest thrill of all.

As great as it was to belong and be physically active and strong, it was also reckless. I was thinking like a healthy person. I was not accepting my limitations. I was not looking ahead to what I could be possibly bringing on to myself. Whilst it was great that I could participate, it probably wasn't wise to participate for the entire game. Moderation was needed if I was to control my lupus and prevent a flare from happening.

As the year rolled on, I continued to battle infections. They were the usual suspects: thrush, bladder infections and heaps of colds. It continued to make battling lupus very challenging. The steroids gave me a lot of energy and eased most of my pain, which enabled me to cope with these infections. But the irony was that these steroids were causing me to be susceptible to catching them in the first place! To have enough energy to concentrate on my schoolwork was a blessing. It really was. I was recovering from a day at school with less fatigue, which was also a vast improvement. I was achieving excellent marks and feedback from my teachers across all of my subjects. I felt encouraged by my progress and my resolve to just keep looking forward and seeing what I could achieve.

* * *

I was under no illusion that suffering from lupus was not all about how it was affecting me. It also deeply affected my immediate family in many intangible ways that are difficult to articulate. For Mum, Dad, Ross and Rebecca, they had to bare witness to my struggle every day. They had to modify their lives and adapt to my needs. Whether it was helping me to have a good rest by being quiet during the afternoon or helping to complete more chores around the house to reduce my household responsibilities, they had to be more accommodating. They had to worry about me in a way that they never had to before. Their hearts had been pulled wide open with feelings of fear and concern for the quality of life I was now experiencing. Whether it be consciously or sub-consciously, they felt helpless in being unable to halt this dreadful disease.

In addition to the worries they already had, the weariness and stress of Mum and Dad's lives became even more challenging when Mum became very ill with a flu-like virus that didn't seem to improve. Over time, it developed into chronic fatigue syndrome; the very disease that I was once thought to be suffering from. It was devastating to see Mum bedridden, fatigued and in pain. Here I was, improving and back at school, and now Mum was also experiencing a chronic illness from which there was no cure or treatment. Only bed rest seemed to help, if at all. Life felt cruel. Devastating. And even sadder.

So, we continued to dig deep as a family, as tough as it was. The blessing of my health improving meant that I was strong enough to help more around the house and to care for Mum. Ross was often not at home so the household jobs were divided mainly between Dad, Rebecca and myself to keep things moving. Rebecca and I managed well with these additional responsibilities. We would often come home from school during the day to prepare lunch for Mum and check in on her when she was particularly unwell. We would sit with Mum, hold her hand and wipe away her tears. We tried to be everything we could be, as loving, giving daughters and now, carers.

* * *

With Mum now ill, the acrimonious relationship with my aunty and granny still continued. It was heartbreaking that they didn't wish to contact Mum to see how she was or how I was. In me and my parents' minds, it was their loss. It was their loss in watching and enjoying the progress I was making in feeling stronger and being able to continue my schooling. This prolonged silence reinforced the fact that as a family, we didn't need anyone to be negative in our lives. We had enough on our plate. If they didn't care to know how I was, well, so be it. I continued to reconcile with myself that I had done nothing wrong.

In many ways, experiencing family discord of this magnitude was an early life lesson in what ignorance was. I was not expecting members of my extended family to be ignorant, uncaring people, but sadly, they were. Maybe their ignorance was born from a place of fear and denial, particularly from my aunty, whom had previously declared that she would resume visiting me only when I was all better. I have no doubt she was simply waiting for my lupus to disappear, and when it did, in her mind, connectedness between our families could be resumed and 'be back to normal'.

What saddens me to this day is the fact that for this disease to happen to me, one that none of us knew too much about at the time, did not evoke any feelings of empathy or an attempt to learn and understand what I was suffering from. Or was it deeper than that? My aunty had reportedly made the comment early on when I first became ill at how disappointing it was, as she had had 'high hopes' for me and what I would achieve in my life. A comment like this implies that my aunty viewed illness in any form as maybe a sign of weakness. That I was no longer worth loving or caring for because she didn't see me as someone worth supporting. It appeared that she had no faith in my ability to rise up to the many challenges lupus was asking me to overcome.

All these years later, it is still difficult to reconcile that their supposed love for me as my aunty and my granny could not enable them to embrace me without prejudice. How sad that they could not reach within themselves to find a way to give me comfort that could have reduced the depth of my suffering. They encountered a disease that they didn't know about nor care to understand. The shallowness of their hearts was on show. But I was learning that this is what ignorance looks like and that it can arise in the most unexpected people and places. It was to be one of my greatest teachers as I grew and moved into an outer world of even greater cruelty than these women had ever shown me.

Chapter Twelve

Under the Radar

When I was in Year 8, before lupus appeared, I was the dark horse of my girls only PE class. Every now and then, our class would complete an activity called the 'Creek Run' as a warm-up. Our high school was built at the end of a dead-end road that backed on to Merri Creek. We would walk out of the school gates, down a sandy path and walk over a short bridge. We would then run a short distance along another sandy walking path along the creek, then run across another bridge that took us over the creek. We would then run along that path; it too, a sandy, walking path that ran along the creek all the way back to the beginning, near our school gates. Basically, it was one big circle. The run took approximately ten minutes to complete.

I remember the first time I ran the Creek Run. In the change rooms prior to the run, all of the trendy, sporty girls who competed in Little Athletics on the weekends tightened the laces of their Nikes and began boasting about how they were going to win the Creek Run. I was in the corner, adjusting my Kmart runners and listening to their bravado. When it came time to line up at the starting line, my heart began thumping. I just wanted to finish with a decent place.

Off we went, and I paced myself nicely during the first part of the run. As the race progressed, I started passing other girls that were ahead of me, one by one. Over the bridge and onto the last part of the Creek Run, I started to gain more speed and more hope in my heart that I could finish the run in a good position. Even more excitingly, as the race progressed, I was gaining speed and catching up to the leader. She just didn't hear me coming as we both rounded the final bend together. Suddenly, I sprinted off, leaving her to catch my dust. It was going to be me. I was going to win the Creek Run! Not one to boast, I was quietly elated as I crossed the finish line. I had beaten the sporty girls, the girls that competed for ribbons and trophies in long-distance running. Me! Though, it was much to the disdain of these girls. Boy, did I cop it in the change room later on. They were furious that I had won. They obviously didn't think I had it in me. But that was, and still is, me – always under the radar.

Being under the radar has actually served me very well in life. Just like the Creek Run, I have always tried to put my head down with minimal fuss and move forward to the best of my ability. I'm always interested to see what could happen, to see what I can achieve. I had often been described as a perfectionist when it came to completing my studies. I hated that term as I did not feel that was me at all. To me, being a perfectionist was someone who was never satisfied with their achievements, no matter how excellent they may be. Someone who was wanting to be 'perfect' at everything they did. Someone who was never happy. That wasn't me at all. I think because I was always a child who was a little too mature, who worried about doing the right thing and who took pride in wanting to do my best, that I was incorrectly labelled with this word.

On many occasions, like the Creek Run, I have surprised myself by what I have been able to do. But having lupus was now changing the way others saw me and what they thought I was now able to achieve. Because of this, every challenge I was greeted with began to feel like a test of how much I was truly accepting that I had an incurable disease. During this time, I felt very proud of how well I was coping with having lupus. I knew I had my limitations. I just didn't want anyone to rule me out, to stop me from trying and reaching for the stars. It mattered so much to me, as I didn't want anyone to take away my hope. Hope was all I had now.

***

As Year 12 progressed, discussion of careers and uni began to take centre stage. For the longest time, ever since I was a little girl, I wanted to become a teacher. I wasn't sure if I wanted to be a primary school teacher or a secondary school teacher, but I knew that teaching was going to be my path. With my lupus diagnosis, this dream was now an uncertainty.

The moment I became a student of my VCE Human Development class, I knew what type of teacher I wanted to be. I wanted to teach VCE Human Development. I absolutely loved this subject. I loved learning about the human body, what impacts on growth and development, about the issues affecting families – simply, all of it. We had an exceptional teacher in Mrs Kerryn Low. She was young, vibrant and extremely dedicated. She worked hard to make our lessons enjoyable, meaningful and memorable. Her approach to teaching inspired me to dream big about becoming a teacher.

I felt much relief knowing that this was what I wanted to do. Striving to pass VCE and succeed in scoring a place at uni, and to study to become a VCE Human Development teacher became my purpose. It gave me much peace knowing that I had a definite plan of what I wished for my life. Unfortunately, not everyone shared my belief in my dream.

'Rachel, I don't think teaching is for you, especially secondary teaching. You are a very quiet, shy girl, and I think that teaching teenagers would be too difficult for you.'

'Rachel, you are simply not well enough to become a teacher, let alone a secondary teacher. It's just not achievable.'

'Rachel, what if you are not well enough to keep up with the job?'

'Teaching is too stressful. You don't need any stress.'

So many comments were made regarding my career choice, but I was insistent on following my dream of becoming a teacher. I hoped that I wasn't being stubborn about it. I really wanted to see if it was possible. I was also of the belief that if I was well enough to work, then shouldn't I be doing something I loved and enjoyed? Wouldn't that be good for my health too?

One of the biggest obstacles was the fact that the only university that offered the teaching course to be able to teach VCE Human Development was a double degree at Deakin Uni's Rusden Campus in Clayton. I would need access to a car to drive over an hour to Rusden, then another hour back home again, if I was to study there. The amount of energy required to attend lectures, tutorials, then the significant travel time, let alone time to study, was huge. It would be an incredible challenge to manage a workload like this and keep my lupus under control.

When it came to pursuing a career, I had only ever envisaged myself teaching. I hoped to become a teacher who treated teaching as a vocation, not a job. I would be dedicated, caring and friendly with my students but also firm and demanding that respect came first. I longed to experience the ability to make a difference in the world. Teaching made this possible. Pursuing studies in Human Development added to this, as I felt excited that I could teach students how to nurture their health and to become more aware of the many social issues affecting the world. This was a subject that mattered and even if they didn't pursue a career in health, students could take the principles of what they were learning into their own lives to practise and even share with others. So many positive outcomes could be achieved.

Even though I was extremely shy when speaking in public, for some reason, I had a strong belief that I would be okay when it came time to stand in front of a class of students. Surprisingly, I never doubted my ability to have the strength and self-esteem needed to be a successful teacher. During this time, I felt frustrated that, unlike so many of my peers, I knew the career path I wished to follow. The negative comments I received about my dream to become a teacher compounded my frustration. I only wished more people could see my potential.

Understandably, my parents were extremely worried about how I would manage completing a course like this, especially so far away from home. After much discussion, they could see that I had my heart set on pursuing teaching and agreed to support me. Ross was looking at buying another car and was prepared to sell me his first car, a Holden Gemini sedan. This was a great solution, as it enabled me to travel all the way to Clayton most days. Being well enough to handle the study load of being a uni student was yet to be seen. My parents and I agreed that if I was successful at being accepted into this course, all I could do was see how I went. If it became too much, then I would have to look at pursuing something else.

Some of my teachers at school were concerned when they learned that I wished to become a teacher. As teachers themselves, they were more than familiar with the stress and demands of the job. They were worried that it would be too much for me. Thankfully, I also had some really encouraging words of support from some of my other teachers. They could see that I had given the prospect of teaching much thought and knew that my conscientious approach to my studies would help me to achieve my teaching goal.

* * *

I felt much comfort from those people who had faith in my teaching capabilities. I really believed that if I was given a chance, I could teach. I knew that it was going to involve hard work. If I was fortunate enough to get into uni, successfully complete my course and gain employment as a teacher, I would be living my life well. For being true to myself, was everything. And in all honesty, I couldn't imagine myself doing anything else with my life.

I continued to persevere with the dual challenges of managing my lupus and completing my VCE. Infections, steroid side-effects and fatigue continued to be my major hurdles health-wise, but with continued support from my family and teachers, I kept getting back up again whenever I was down and unwell. The enormity of completing my VCE was not lost on me, as it was for so many of my peers, and I continued to find it very difficult to integrate myself into their world, when all I continued to hear was how easily life was unfolding for them.

As exams approached, I became very anxious about how I would cope. I absolutely hated exams and I was very scared that I wouldn't be able to remember everything I needed to. I continued to find writing by hand painful. Even though I knew that I could be granted extra writing time during the exams if I needed it, I was still fraught with worry about whether I could perform well under this pressure. I was also very worried about suffering a lupus flare during the middle of the exams. If that was the case, I wouldn't be able to take the exams and would achieve a mock score based on my achievements in VCE thus far. Thankfully, I had achieved excellent results for each of the CATS that I had submitted throughout the year and I was so grateful, for if I didn't perform as well on my exams, I had high marks to counteract any low scores. But I was still agonising over the possibility of being unwell during this time. There was a lot buzzing around in my head.

I was experiencing much stress at this time, but with much support from my family, I was reminded that I had already achieved much to be proud of by simply being well enough to attend school and to participate in my VCE classes. All I could do was to try my very best in preparing for the exams and the results I achieved would take care of themselves. Whatever that was meant to be would be.

When exam time came around, I was amazed at the good health I was experiencing. I took good care of myself and worked through each exam, one step at a time. I managed to complete most of the exams within the required time. It was hard, but I got there! When each of my exams was completed, the relief was immense. However, this feeling of elation was short-lived, as I replaced the anxiety of completing my exams with the anxiety of being able to achieve the score that I needed to be accepted into my chosen course at uni. Two long, agonizing periods of waiting were on their way: the wait for exam scores and the wait for uni acceptance. It was going to be tough.

As Year 12 came to an end, remarkably, a wonderful, unexpected honour was awarded to me during the long wait for exam scores to be announced. I received the Caltex Award. An actual award! In fact, it was a beautiful medal. Year 12 teachers were asked to select one student in Year 12 to receive the Caltex medal. The award was to be given to a student who had achieved consistently high results throughout the year and had worked conscientiously. It was the first time the school had been given the Caltex Award to recognise student achievement and I was the first recipient – amazing! It was such a wonderful surprise. I was so overcome with emotion at receiving this special award. It was like a bright light of shiny stars sparkling through me, whispering, 'Rachel, well done, girl. You are on the right track.'

The best thing about receiving this award was how proud my parents were. They were really thrilled that my efforts and achievements had been recognised in this way. It was such a positive end to a difficult secondary school experience for me. To this day, I still feel emotional when I remember receiving this award and the symbolism of perseverance that it represents. I cherish it very much.

Pleasingly and reassuringly, I achieved a very good result for my VCE. While I didn't perform as well on my exams, I managed to achieve a score that would give me a chance of being selected to my chosen course at uni. The wait after Christmas for uni entry results was agonising. I did not cope well at all. I was still so worried that I wouldn't be selected, and if I didn't, what would I do if I couldn't become a Human Development teacher? I was in knots. Somehow, I managed to relax and enjoy the rewards of completing my VCE studies by having a good break, but I was easily agitated and had a few teary meltdowns along the way (thank you, Mum and Dad, for always picking me up and putting me back together again).

When I received the letter from Deakin Uni to say that I had been successful in being accepted into the Double Degree of Bachelor of Secondary Teaching and Bachelor of Consumer Science, I was rapt. Elated! Relieved! *Ahh!* I was in. I was going to learn how to be a teacher! It was such an exciting time. I was one of few students in Year 12 at my school to be accepted into uni, which reminded me how fortunate I was. It was such an amazing achievement for me on so many levels. For the years of struggling with ill health, it was a moment where I could lament on the pain and frustration I had endured during secondary school and truly enjoy the feeling of being successful, particularly when so many people didn't believe that I would be well enough to finish school, let alone be accepted into uni.

Staying 'under the radar' gave me strength, as I was able to chip away at all of the work that was required, without too many high expectations from others. It was also momentous to me because my achievement was equally joyous for my parents. They were integral in giving me the opportunity and faith in myself to pursue my dreams. They had walked through every challenging moment with me. All the years of doubt, fear and worry had culminated in a moment where I had achieved the supposed 'unachievable'. My teachers were also experiencing the happiness of seeing my goals coming to life. They had supported me and shown compassion and understanding in trying to relieve the stresses associated with completing VCE as a sick student. The support services that my situation had helped to develop were now in place for future students who would need the support that I had in completing their VCE. That was a very positive outcome indeed.

Whilst my success in achieving a place at uni was extremely gratifying, my experience in the uni world would continue to test and shape me, through a multitude of more unexpected challenges I had to face. This has since given me the foundation of resilience from which I continue to grow.

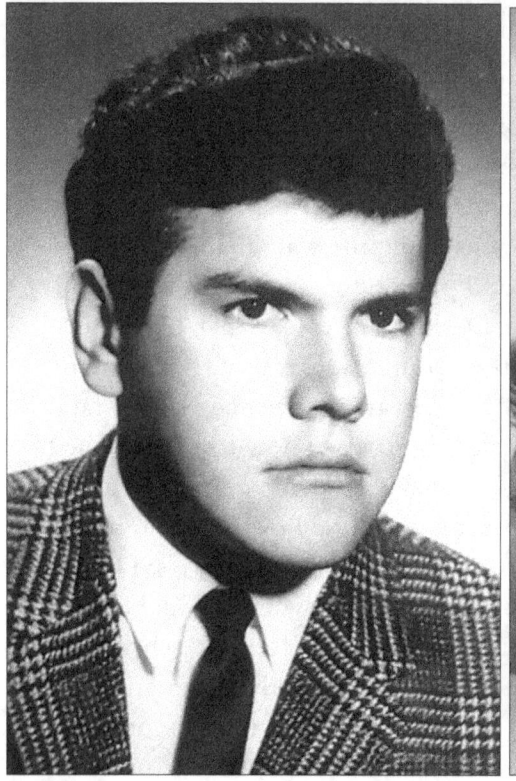
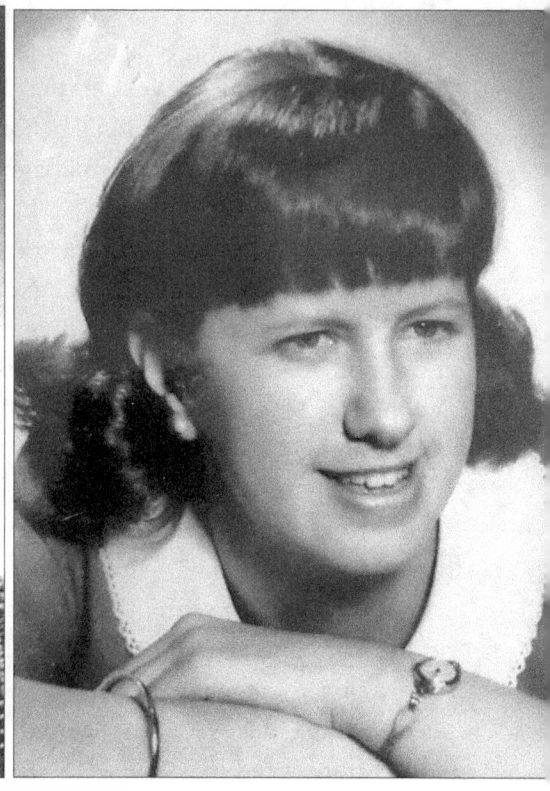

Top left and right: Dad, 21, and Mum, 17, in 1968 during the early days of their courtship.

Left: A quiet moment of me, aged 4, playing at Greenbrook kindergarten in 1980.

Right: Me – being a typical, cheeky 2 year old, 1977.

Right: Ross, 10, Bec, 5, and me, 8, ready to leave for our pa's 79th birthday – 1983.

Below: Ross, 7, our grandma Lea (from Darwin), Bec, 2, and me, 5, in our lounge room, Epping 1981.

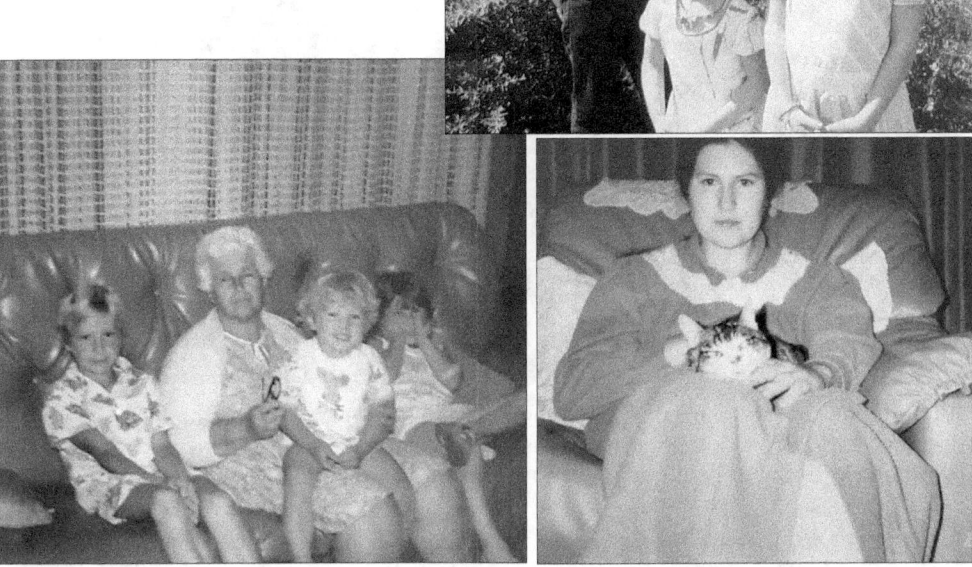

Middle right: Gypsy and me, 15. We were both sick at the time. I lived in this dressing gown and missed the majority of Year 10 due to being ill with undiagnosed lupus.

Below left: I painted this tree when I was 10 years old. It is a copy of an original painted by my pa, who loved to paint. I hope to one day return to drawing and painting.

Below right: At the beginning of Year 10, 1991. I fell ill not long after this picture was taken and did not return to school until the remaining few weeks of the year.

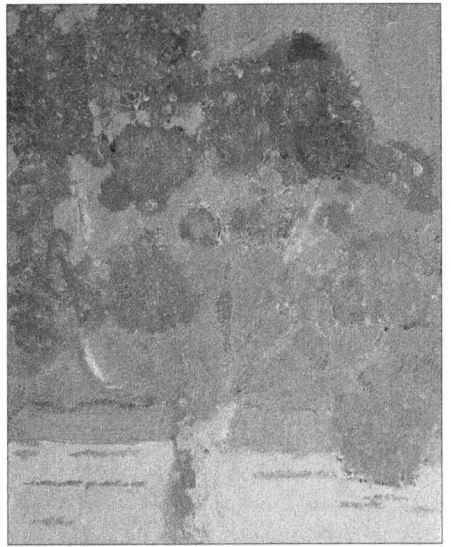
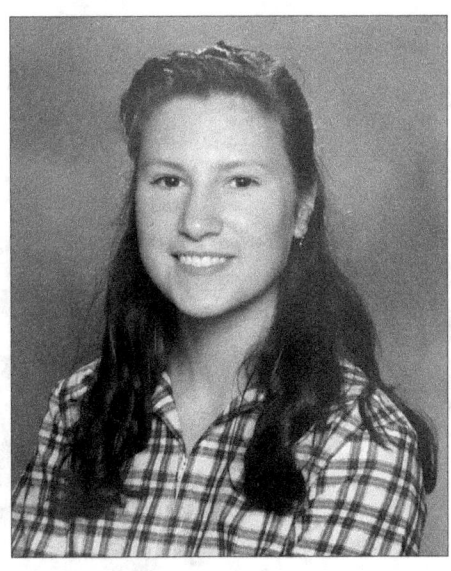

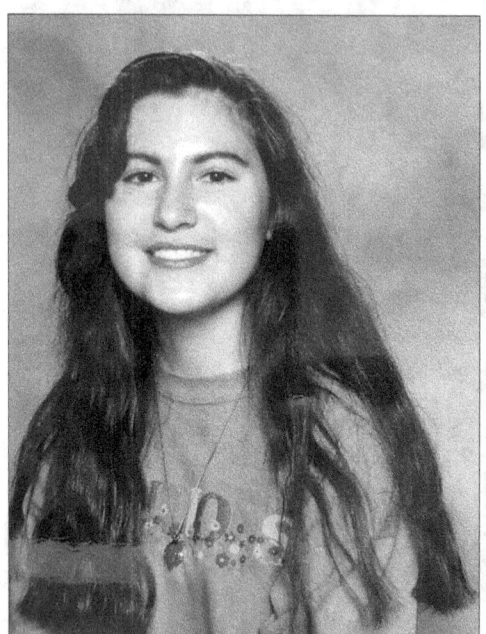 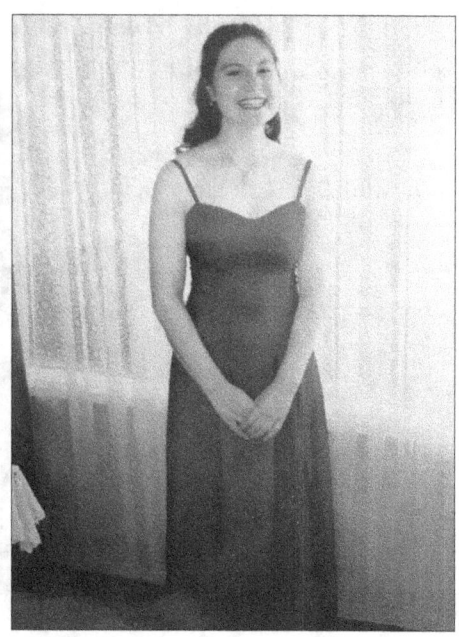

Top left: Back at school for the beginning of Year 11 in 1992. I was bloated from steroid use but feeling more energetic and in less pain. What a difference in my appearance compared with the previous year's school photo!

Top right: Ready to leave for my Year 12 school formal. I remember feeling so thrilled that I was feeling well and able to successfully complete the end of this huge school year.

Bottom left: My former teacher and now friend, Karen Bryce, and me at my Year 12 school formal. Karen has been a wonderful support to me over the years.

Bottom right: One of so many moments during my time as a uni student – busy, hard at work at the dining table at home.

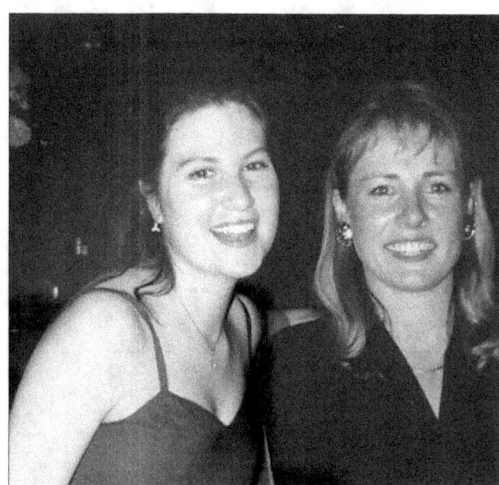 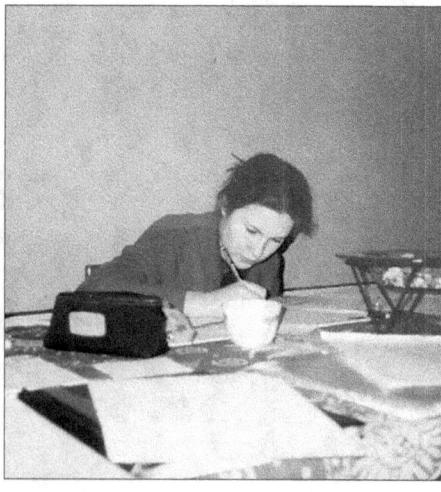

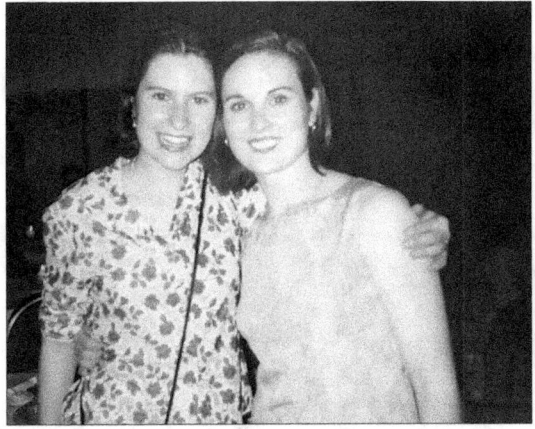
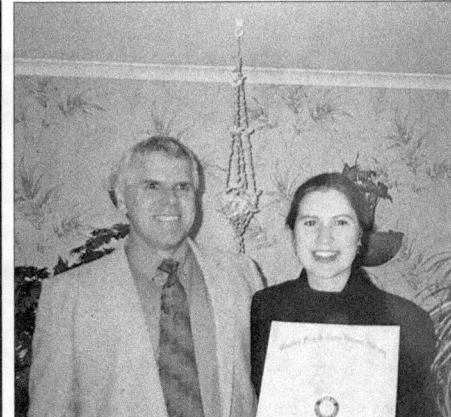

Top Left: My dear friend Jackie Maartensz (nee Orwin) and me, 21 years old, at her 21st birthday party in 1996. We met during a group assignment at uni and have been friends ever since!

Top Right: Dad and me, aged 22, after our return home from a Deakin University award ceremony, where I was awarded membership of the 'Golden Key National Honour Society' in 1997 in recognition of Outstanding Scholastic Achievement and Excellence. I was stoked to receive this!

Right: Aunty Bron, Uncle Fred and me after I had received the award for 'Outstanding Student in Studies in Teaching Home Economics' at the award ceremony at Deakin University. Sadly, Uncle Fred passed away from Alzheimer's disease in 2018.

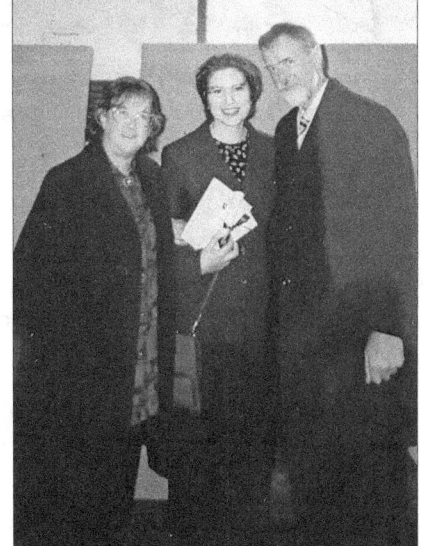

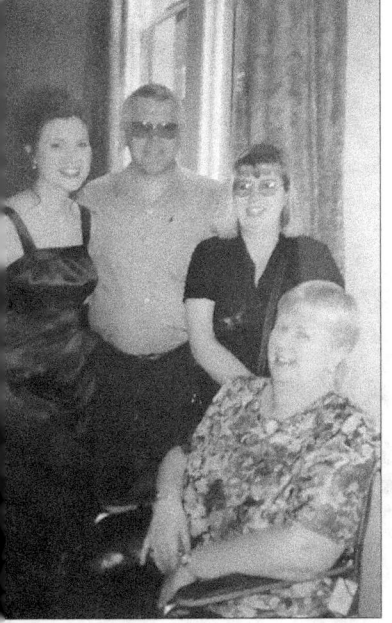

Left: My Dad, Bec, Mum and me, aged 20. I was a bridesmaid for my friend Marjolijn. It was lovely for my family to be there and particularly Mum, to be well enough to attend the service.

Right: Me at my 21st birthday, 1996, held at a theatre restaurant in the city. I celebrated with a group of uni friends. I felt happy and well, not long after my breast lump was removed. It was a great night!

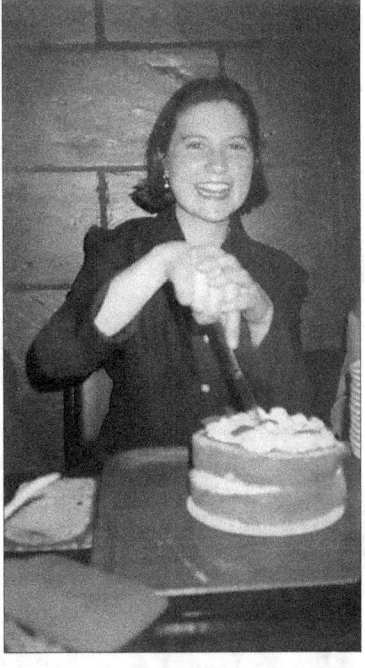

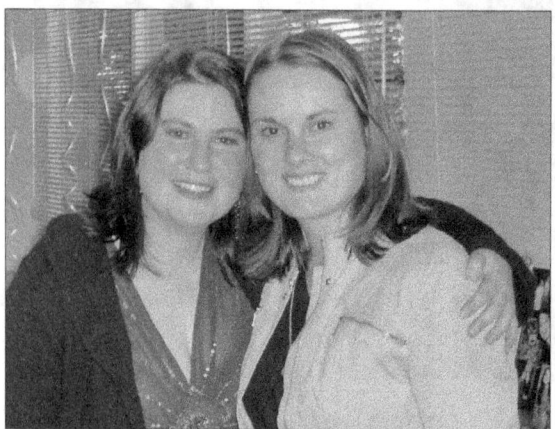 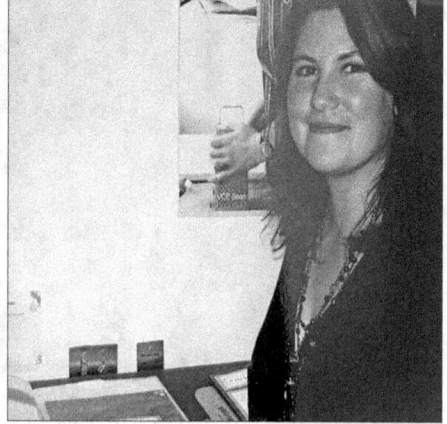

Top left: Jackie and me at my 30th birthday celebration, 2005. I was very ill during this time – my lupus rash/fever was constant, and I had gained weight and was extremely bloated due to significantly higher doses of steroids and methotrexate to keep my lupus under control.

Top right: Attending the opening night of the VCE Season of Excellence 2006 Top Designs at Melbourne Museum. Two of my Year 12 Food Technology students had their folios displayed in this exhibition – as their teacher, I was so proud of their achievements (another one of my students also had their folio displayed in the same exhibition in 2007). I was extremely ill during this time and I collapsed three months later – too ill to work for eighteen months.

Bottom left: Graduation day! I received a double degree – Bachelor in Teaching (Secondary) and Bachelor in Applied Science – in 1998. A momentous, emotional achievement for me.

Bottom right: My beautiful friend, Maree Pell, and me at a function for her retirement from teaching. She was an inspirational teacher and a loving, supportive friend to me. Sadly, she passed away from secondary breast cancer in 2012.

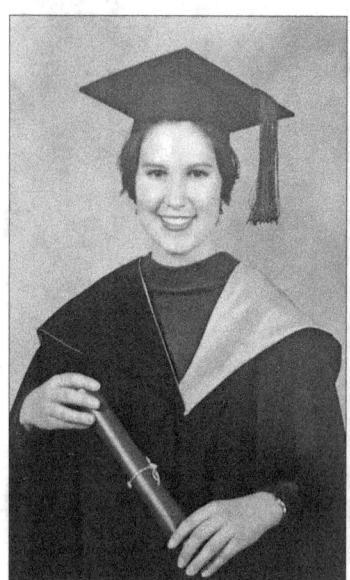 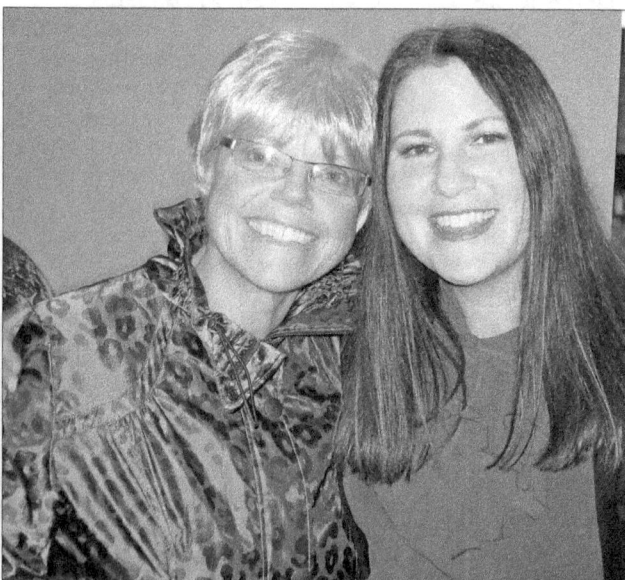

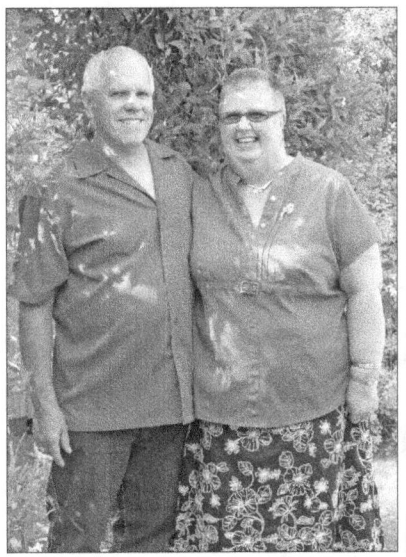
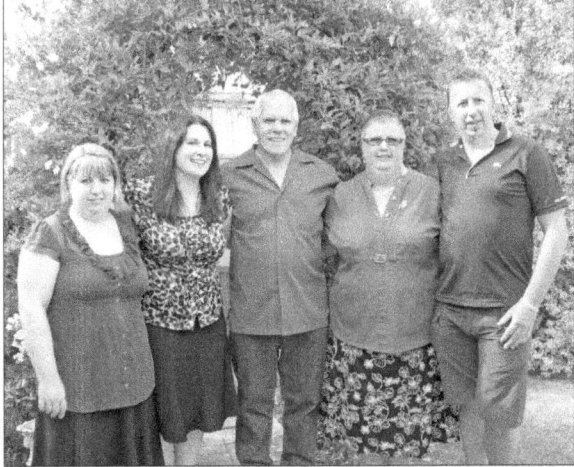

Top left and top right: Mum, Dad, Bec, Ross and me at Mum and Dad's 40th wedding anniversary celebration in 2011. We celebrated this special occasion with an afternoon tea at their home with close friends and family. It was wonderful to see Mum and Dad being celebrated with much love after years of many family challenges.

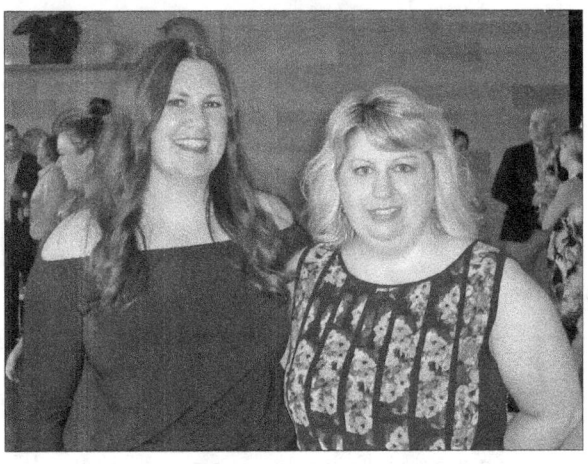

Middle right: My gorgeous sister, Bec, and me at Ross and Naomi's wedding in January 2016. Unfortunately, I was battling another nasty lupus flare, which had resulted in more steroids and weight gain. I was struggling to keep my lupus under control, and I collapsed five months after the wedding.

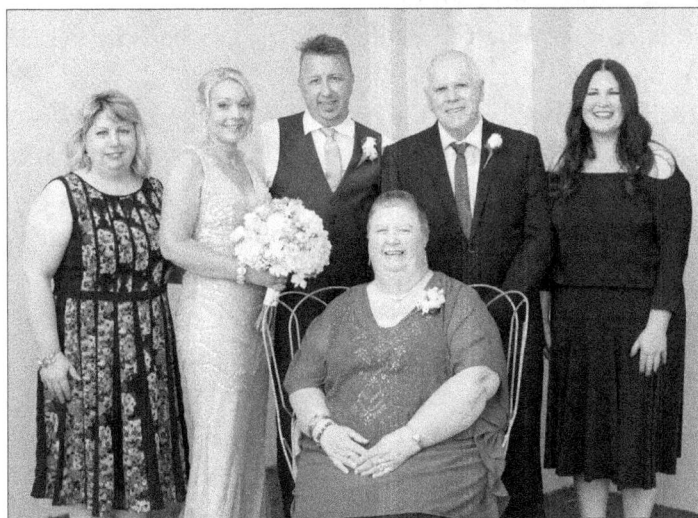

Above: Family portrait of Bec, my sister-in-law Naomi, Ross, Dad, myself and Mum on Ross and Naomi's wedding day – January, 2016.

Chapter Thirteen

Clipped Wings

I began studying at Deakin Uni at its Rusden Campus in Clayton, in the summer of 1994. The problem of how I would travel to uni each day had been solved. I had purchased Ross' car, the 1984 Gemini, with my savings and some help from Mum and Dad. Even though it had been Ross' car, I was so excited that it had now become mine. I had my very own car! How grown-up was I? I felt so happy.

Travelling to uni each day proved quite the adventure. I had grown up in the outer northern suburbs of Melbourne and was only familiar with that side of town. Dad had taught me to drive in the family car, a manual column shift Mitsubishi Express seven-seater van. He had taught me to drive along many long, treacherous country roads when I was on my learner's permit and it had served me well in learning how to drive across Melbourne in busy, unfamiliar traffic. I had completed a couple of practise drives prior to the orientation programme at uni and I coped very well.

It was both an exciting and anxious time beginning life as a uni student. For the first time since attending kindergarten, I didn't know anybody. It was a clean slate. Nobody knew I was sick. They didn't know I had lupus. I felt normal and enjoyed blending in with everyone else, as they were equally as nervous as I was about the impending uni life that lay ahead.

As the course was a double degree to become primarily a Human Development teacher, it also incorporated many nutrition and cooking classes that would allow students to also be able to teach Food Technology in secondary schools. The title of Home Economics teacher was being phased out during this time, but traditionally, teachers in secondary schools at this time would have completed a Home Economics degree that enabled them to teach Food Technology, Human Development and even Health Education. Teachers of these subjects had been traditionally female and my course was no different. The only male students I encountered in my classes were in my teaching classes.

The girls I met came, predominantly, from the south-eastern suburbs of Melbourne. None from the west or the north like me. Most of them had been educated in the private school system. Compared with me, they seemed so confident and experienced at life. Even though it was a teaching degree, most of the girls I met were not sure if being a teacher was going to be their path in life. They were just biding time, enjoying the prospect of uni life, part-time work and the freedoms of socialising that came with it.

I embraced the routine of uni life very quickly, which was a real surprise to me, given my shyness and fear of being out of my comfort zone. I loved sitting in the lecture theatre, listening and learning about topics that interested me. Even more, I loved sitting down in the cafeteria eating bowls of hot chips with new student friends I was quickly making, as we waited between classes. Walking to class and seeing bands perform live was new and exhilarating. The energy and buzz of uni life was something to behold. I was grateful for every bit of it, particularly as I was the first child on my mother's side of the family to attend uni.

I was also thankful for my ability to cope with the demands of being a uni student. I was well enough to be up very early to make the drive across town to be seated at many an 8 am lecture and leave at around 3 or 4 pm most days. Friday was uni-free which enabled me to rest and recover, in addition to the weekend, and to study and begin completing the many assignments that were quickly piling up. My regime of steroids, anti-inflammatories and the anti-malarial drug hydroxychloroquine, also known as called Plaquenil, gave me the energy and strength I needed to fulfil this role. My lupus was being well-controlled and symptoms were minimal. It felt like I had been given wings and I was starting to fly.

LUPUS = *Lift Up, Persevere, Use Strength*

* * *

I wasn't flying high for long, as my wings were clipped one rainy night on the drive home from campus. I was sitting in the middle of the intersection of Waterdale Road and Bell Street in West Heidelberg, waiting to complete a right-hand turn. Chocolate Starfish was booming through my radio speakers, the car window wipers clearing the downpour of rain with their rhythmic movement. Safe to turn, I started to steer right and accelerate when, suddenly, in the darkness, I heard a long, piercing screech of car brakes. Moving towards me at a speed I had never felt before was another car. In less than a second, I glimpsed the frightened faces of its passengers behind its jutting windowpanes, for the impact, the sound and the movement of my car spinning had enveloped me completely. All I could do was hit the brakes and hold on. It felt like everything was happening in slow motion. It was incomprehensible. My brain had trouble understanding what was happening to me.

When the sensation of tumbling and spinning ceased, the sound and vision of shattering glass and someone trying to open my driver's side door filled my conscious state. A large, middle-aged woman had managed to open my door. She had taken hold of me and was trying to hug me, reassuring me that I was okay. She said that she had seen everything and that I had done nothing wrong. Another man appeared, uttering the same words. I was mute. I was staring at them, unable to speak. They shoved a piece of paper in my hand and told me that they couldn't stay but they were happy to be my witnesses and told me to ring them. And then they disappeared into the night.

What on earth had happened? One minute I was singing along to the radio, safe to turn into Waterdale Road and the next minute, I was trapped inside a terrifying vortex of insurmountable speed and confusion.

I was only just coming to my senses and realising that I had been in a car accident when moments after the kind woman and young man had disappeared, my driver's side door was pulled wide open and a middle-aged man was furiously screaming at me, 'What have you done?' His wife was shrieking repeatedly in their car, which was now stationary and opposite mine, in the middle of the intersection. I was confused. Mortified. What had I done? What did he mean? I had no time to respond when another man appeared and asked the angry man to step aside and leave me alone. Thankfully, he did just that but his verbal abuse and tirade did not diminish as he continued to accuse me of deliberately hitting their car. At the insistence of this strange but helpful man, he eventually walked away and I was able to feel a little safer.

The man who had intervened and defended me then squatted down to my level, as I sat shaking, covered in shards of glass in my driver's seat. He checked to see if I was injured. Miraculously, it appeared that I wasn't. A number of huge, sharp and jagged shards of glass were just sitting on top of me – no blood in sight, no scratches to be seen. My seat belt had kept me firmly in my seat. The left side of my car was all squashed up and the roof on the left-side front seat was so close to me, it was touching my head.

The man was an ambulance driver and he began to explain to me what had happened. He and his fellow paramedic had to urgently attend to their patient who was travelling in their van, which meant that they had to stop the ambulance in the middle of a right-hand slip lane that happened to be in the opposite part of the intersection to where my car was. Realising that the ambulance was not moving, the driver of the car behind the stationary ambulance grew impatient, and upon a green light, he quickly pulled out from behind the ambulance and accelerated into the intersection to make a right turn. At this stage, I was already in the middle of completing a right-hand turn. At that moment in time, it was safe and clear for me to do so. He collided with the left side of my car at such a force that my car spun around in a complete circle.

The police arrived very quickly to the scene, as their headquarters were stationed on the corner of Waterdale Road and Bell Street. The ambulance driver needed to return to assist his patient but I saw that he briefly spoke to the police officers to establish his version of events. The two police officers in attendance also checked to see if I was alright. They then needed to attend to the driver of the car that had hit me and instruct him to calm down, as he had returned to my car again and reignited his abusive attack on me. In that moment, I felt so traumatised. So vulnerable. So alone.

After a short time, I managed to feel more lucid, more able to comprehend what was being said to me. A tow truck had arrived to take my car away. My new car. My very own car. I had been driving my new car for only three weeks. Three weeks and it had all come, literally, to a screaming halt. Even though the police officers had spoken to the ambulance driver, the position of my car in the intersection indicated that

I had not given way to traffic on my right. The police officers needed to get a statement of my version of events, so I had to go to the police station with them. I had no choice. I looked around at my belongings that had been flung around the interior of my car. Complete chaos. I slowly picked up everything I could see and gingerly climbed out of my car. I'm sure I cut a solemn figure, clutching my uni papers, textbooks, handbag, Melways and my club steering lock, as I watched the tow truck drivers hoist my much loved, damaged car onto their truck. I was just eighteen years old.

I walked to the police station with the officers and gave them my statement. I gave them the number of the witnesses who had reassured me that I was not in the wrong. Thankfully, they were very kind and showed me much compassion with the situation I found myself in. They asked me if I would like a lift home. I imagined the look of panic and confusion a visit from two police officers would illicit from my parents and politely declined. I put them through enough worry on a daily basis and didn't wish for them to be given a fright. What had happened was already going to be a significant event for them to overcome as parents.

Coincidently, family friends of ours lived further down Waterdale Road in Ivanhoe. I asked if it was possible for the police officers to drop me off at their house instead. They were happy to oblige. The shocked sight of me walking up their garden path with a police officer while holding onto all of my belongings was enough of a shock for my friends to comprehend, let alone my parents seeing me like this. They rang my parents and told them what had happened, reassuring them that I was fine. I wasn't speaking much. Monosyllabic answers were all I could manage. I hadn't even shed a tear.

Dad and Ross came to pick me up soon after. They looked lost for words and very distraught at what had happened. When we arrived home and I walked in the door, tears came tumbling down my face. I was so relieved to be home. Safe. The floodgates of shock and trauma had been opened and I sobbed and sobbed. I was inconsolable. I felt so confused. Even though I had been reassured that the car accident wasn't my fault, I still felt responsible. My parents had given me so much in helping me to have my own car. They had paid for my driving lessons, my license application and now, after only three weeks of driving, it was all over. I was bereft. I felt like I had let them down. I had gone from feeling content at being well enough to attend uni and to be able to drive the long distance it demanded, to not knowing what was going to happen to me. How was I going to get to classes now?

The next day, Dad told me gently that it was important that I get back on the horse, so to speak. He said that it was really important for my confidence that I sit behind the wheel and go for a drive. Begrudgingly, I buckled up in the old Mitsubishi Express and did just that. And I was glad that I did. Dad was right. To be back in the driver's seat helped me to feel competent about my driving skills and reduced my fear of driving.

A visit to the car repair shop concluded that my Holden Gemini was indeed a write-off. It could not be salvaged. I was devastated. I loved driving my new car. It made me feel independent and free. And now that experience of driving to campus each day appeared to be over before it truly began. I felt angry. Cheated. It felt like everything in my life was always so bloody hard.

Thankfully, I was not found guilty of reckless driving. The woman and young man, her son, proved to be true to their word, and their witness statements of what had happened, along with those of the ambulance driver, cleared me of any wrongdoing. I was so relieved. I couldn't express in words how relieved I truly was. The thought of causing harm to anyone is extremely distressing to me. Thankfully, the driver of the other car and his wife were not injured.

Aside from the relief of not being the cause of the accident, it started to sink in, what a miracle it was that I was not seriously injured or killed. Worse, that if I had a passenger in the front seat, they would definitely be seriously injured or possibly killed. I would constantly stop and reflect on the accident and the amazement that I did not have a single scratch on me. How extraordinary that the huge shards of glass that fell from the car windows, simply landed on me as though someone had gently placed them there. The sheer force of impact should have resulted in some type of injury for me. It was as if during the time that the car was spinning, I had been wrapped up in a protective bubble. Maybe I had angels taking care of me in that moment. I certainly hope so. My gratitude for being alive was immense and the what-if scenarios would frequently play over in my mind. The post-trauma of the accident was ongoing for a very long time after the accident. Every time I heard the brakes of a car or a loud noise, my heart would beat out of my chest and I was immediately back in my Gemini, spinning out of control. I just had to ride it out during moments like these and take one step at a time.

* * *

After much discussion about how I was going to make it to uni each day, my parents had decided to reach out to Mum's brother and his wife, Uncle Fred and Aunty Bron. They lived with their children, Martin and Megan, in East Bentleigh, an hour away in Melbourne's south-eastern suburbs and not far from Deakin Uni's campus. On the phone, Mum told Uncle Fred and Aunty Bron about my accident and how it was now going to affect my ability to attend uni via car each day. Mum asked them if it was possible for me to live with them for a short while during the week so I could attend classes. They said that they were more than happy to help and would love to have me come and stay.

We rarely saw them while we were growing up and I didn't know them very well at all. I felt anxious about being a new member of their family, but I needn't have been. They were extremely welcoming and made me feel at home straight away. We worked out that Dad would drive me down to their house on Sunday night. I would stay until Thursday night, when Dad would come and pick me up to take me home again. I would catch the bus to campus each day. It was all quite overwhelming. New to attending uni on the other side of town, experiencing the trauma of my car accident, living with a new family and navigating the bus in suburbs I was unfamiliar with; it was so much change in such a short span of time. I was overwhelmed.

* * *

The impact of my car accident was of great concern to my parents and my rheumatologist. I was at risk of suffering from a major lupus flare due to the emotional stress of the car accident. To prevent a lupus flare, I was instructed to increase my steroid intake. This helped so much. The steroids gave me extra energy to cope with all of the changes that were happening in my life. For me, whenever I suffered a lupus flare, I would become severely fatigued, and pain in my shoulder joints and upper back would intensify, my thighs would feel muscularly sore, heavy and painful, I would have a headache and fever, my breathing would become laboured and shallow, and I would be in bed for days on end, sleeping when not awake from the pain. An increase of steroids enabled the symptoms of the lupus flare to settle.

As steroids are an immunosuppressant medication, it is their job to attack the disease and shut down the symptoms that are escalating in my body. It is quite the miracle drug. After increasing my steroid dose, symptoms would diminish after a short while. It would depend on the severity of the flare as to how long this would take. Sometimes it took a couple of days, other times a week or more. I knew that I was improving when more energy and strength returned and my pain subsided. The pain in my hands, however, would still remain.

Once my lupus flare symptoms had subsided, I would then begin the long journey of tapering off my high steroid dose. Learning to live with and manage my lupus soon felt like a game of Snakes and Ladders. It's the only way I can describe this to people, because I have had so many times in my life where I have been managing my lupus really well and then, all of a sudden, a stressful event would occur or worse, where there appeared to be no reason at all for a flare of my symptoms to occur. I could be climbing along each rung of the ladder, moving forward slowly but assuredly each day and then, *bang*, my dice would fall on a slithering snake and I would slide all the way down to the bottom of the board. I would then have to find the strength via steroids and positive will to pick myself back up and begin the slow path up the board and onto those ladder rungs again, hoping that I never land on another snake.

* * *

During this time, I was also learning that my lupus symptoms were slightly changing. Whilst I knew I was sensitive to the sun, I didn't know how severely until the day I went to the footy with Ross and Rebecca. We were at the MCG (Melbourne Cricket Ground) for an afternoon match. It was a mild, sunny day. We were seated in the middle of the stands, in direct line of the sun's warm rays. By the time the match was over and we were in the car to go home, I was feeling sick. My face looked red and sunburnt, my lupus butterfly rash spread right across my cheeks. I had the chills, a blinding headache and all I wanted to do was lay down. I spread myself out (strapped in, of course) on the back seat of Ross' car. My symptoms then worsened. All of the classic lupus flare symptoms that I experienced appeared and I was in a serious flare for a couple of weeks. How frightening. A beautiful sunny day at the MCG to enjoy the footy, had made me very ill. Gee, this disease was cruel. Sadly, that was the last time I went to the footy during the day. I have only ever attended AFL games at night, safe from the harsh, dangerous rays of the sun.

I have often been gobsmacked when people have had the nerve to ask me what I have done to cause a lupus flare. And many people have done so over the years. The flare I had after going to the footy was, I guess, something I had unintentionally caused. Being accused of making myself ill is always upsetting. I guess people are implying that I am not resting enough or looking after myself properly. For someone to imply that there is a specific trigger within my behaviour that can result in a flare is so insulting in itself, particularly when I think of the many sacrifices Lupus Warriors such as myself have to make each day in order to combat symptoms of the disease the best way we can. It is always so rude and it gets me quite angry when I am asked this question. It speaks of ignorance and insensitivity.

The best answer I have always given is this, 'I suffer from a chronic, incurable disease. It gets to do what it likes, when it likes. I can only do so much.' That seems to shut them up! To be honest, it is upsetting that I even have to defend myself in the first place. I take comfort that I am not alone, that Lupus Warriors all over the world also endure this level of questioning – as would people with all sorts of chronic, invisible autoimmune diseases. What we need is change. Greater education and awareness of lupus may stop this question from being asked at all.

* * *

Experiencing the terror of this car accident was extremely humbling. Going through the trauma of this experience, it became clear to me that just because I was battling this beastly disease, I was not immune from the frailties of life. I was not a protected species. Life wasn't saying, 'There, there, Rachel. You are battling lupus. You have got enough on your plate. We will leave you alone and not add to your long list of challenges.' It was saying, 'Yes, life is going be tough, but you know this already, so keep doing your best when the hits come. And they will.' And they have. The hits have kept on coming.

Chapter Fourteen

Plodding Along

A few months after my car accident, my parents informed me that they were planning to sell our family piano to Aunty Bron and Uncle Fred as a means of finding the money to buy me a car. My cousin Megan was a budding piano player and could benefit from having the piano to practise on. No one in our family played the piano. It served as a beautiful piece of furniture in our loungeroom and a lovely resting place for family photos. I was quite emotional about the prospect of Mum and Dad selling the piano. Dad had bought the piano for Mum who wanted to start playing it again when they were newly married. It had such sentimental meaning for them both. Additionally, it was a reminder of Pa, who had passed away when I was nine years old and had often played the piano when he visited us as children.

I was distraught that Mum and Dad would do this for me. Again, I felt responsible. But I also felt very loved. My parents were prepared to sacrifice their piano to help me fulfil my dream of becoming a teacher. They reassured me that it was fine. It was the only way that I was able to have money to purchase a car, given that I wasn't well enough to work part-time and save for one myself.

Whilst I had been managing quite well travelling to campus via the bus, and sometimes being dropped home to Aunty Bron and Uncle Fred's by a friend from uni who happened to live a few streets away, Mum and Dad felt that having a car would help me to manage my lupus with more independence. For example, if I was feeling unwell at uni, I could leave and drive home without having to wait for the bus. Staying with Aunty Bron and Uncle Fred during the week was working out so well that they offered to continue this arrangement until I finished my double degree, which all going to plan, would take four years. That way, I could stay with them a couple of nights during the week, to reduce the impact of a draining two hours' drive each day. This arrangement aimed to hopefully help me to conserve more energy and maintain my health.

Uncle Fred was great with cars and offered to help me buy one through the trading post. For the price of $1,500, we found a lovely manual Toyota Corolla sedan, 1977 edition. It was a brown-mustard colour but somehow still appealing! And it was going to be my car. It was such a special gift that Mum and Dad were giving me and I felt the responsibility of taking care of this vehicle very seriously. We had not been raised as spoiled or entitled kids, but with my lupus battle and the nasty car accident I had experienced, the fragility of life was clearly imprinted on everything I had. I wanted so much to respect the generosity and sacrifice my parents were making for me. I felt so fortunate to have another opportunity to drive my own car. I prayed and prayed that I wouldn't have another car accident. I hoped that the days ahead would be a little brighter and I looked forward to many happy drives in my new car.

For me, seeing our family piano sitting in Aunty Bron and Uncle Fred's dining room was very difficult. It was a constant reminder of what my parents had given up for me. Whenever I was staying there, I couldn't look at it and I would try to pretend it wasn't there. It was, however, lovely to see Megan enjoying it and playing it regularly.

As my life as a uni student progressed, I would drive my Corolla to uni from my family home and then stay at Aunty Bron and Uncle Fred's for a day or two, and be back home again on weekends and during days off from uni. I felt so happy. I was enjoying uni and the independence that driving gave me. My parents continued to be so generous, giving me money for petrol, stationery and enough left over for hot chips at the campus cafeteria. It was to be treasured, as I did not wish to waste a single cent. It was financially challenging for Mum and Dad to support me in this way. It was not lost on me how lucky I was to be able to fulfil life as a uni student, albeit differently from those I knew at uni. My depth of gratitude for what my parents were able to give me was profound.

Additionally, the generosity of Aunty Bron and Uncle Fred in welcoming me into their home, giving me shelter and keeping me fed, loved and cared for, was also incredibly humbling. It embedded in me a maturity that was of stark difference to my friends at uni. They were all working, studying and socialising to the hilt. It was all so easy for them. Not being well enough to have a part-time job set me apart from my uni friends. I continued to find ways of concealing my illness where possible. Whilst I didn't feel it was because I was ashamed that I was ill or that I was angry that lupus had happened to me, I simply enjoyed blending in like everyone else. It meant that I didn't have to draw any extra attention to myself or to the fact that I wasn't working like they were. Being under the radar was my modus operandi. When the subject of work did come up, I felt shy and a little awkward, having to find ways to explain why I wasn't able to work part-time or go to nightclubs every weekend as they did.

Over time, as I formed closer friendships at uni, I was able to explain that I suffered from lupus with more ease and that this was the reason why I was unable to work and study at the same time. But I found it difficult when I was in group situations. I would do anything not to be the centre of attention. Lupus continued to challenge my shyness. Whether I liked it or not, lupus was trying to lift me out of my shell, teaching me to feel more comfortable in opening up and talking about myself. But I continued to feel very resentful about this.

Managing my lupus at uni meant that I had to have a nap every day in the afternoon. I would find sitting through lectures and tutorials quite draining. A daily rest was critical to the successful management of preventing lupus flares where possible. As time went on, I started to have low blood pressure and I would often nearly pass out and faint. I learnt breathing strategies and would use them if I came close to fainting, which helped. But these episodes could come on so quickly and prove to be an additional symptom to be mindful of and to prevent where possible.

I was still vulnerable to infections but not as severely as I was during my VCE years, as I was on a more steady, lower dose of steroids. Steroids continued to be my best friend. They gave me life. They helped me to participate in the world. But they were also going to be my enemy over time. Their immediate side effects, such as weight gain, bloating and mood swings continued to be present. However, the threat of developing the bone condition, osteoporosis, as a result of long-term steroid use, continued to be very real. I needed to go to the Austin Hospital for regular bone scans to ensure that my bone density was in the healthy range. Calcium supplements in addition to a dairy-enriched diet and exercise where possible would also help to prevent the threat of developing osteoporosis.

Plaquenil, the hydroxychloroquine anti-malaria medication I was taking, was also a possible enemy. Its job was to reduce inflammation in my body. But over time, it had the ability to ruin my eyesight. It could cause cataracts and I needed to see an ophthalmologist twice a year to ensure the quality of my vision remained unaffected. If there were signs of damage to my eyes, I would have to stop taking Plaquenil immediately. Amazingly, I have been taking the medication for twenty-seven years and thankfully, so far so good.

In regard to the cause of the mysterious swelling, pain and coldness in my hands, my new rheumatologist, who I began seeing after my time at the Royal Children's Hospital, diagnosed my condition immediately. I was suffering from Raynaud's phenomenon. The condition causes some areas of the body – such as your fingers and toes – to feel numb and cold in response to cold temperatures or stress. In Raynaud's phenomenon, smaller arteries that supply blood to the skin become narrow, thus limiting blood circulation to affected areas.[16] This was causing my pain and the coldness in my hands. As you can imagine, it was a relief to finally have my pain and symptoms diagnosed.

Taking my medication regularly, napping each day, early nights, limiting stress and keeping socialising to a bare minimum were the keys to managing life with lupus as a uni student. The pace of attending lectures and tutorials and the time needed to complete the myriad of assignments was demanding for me. But I was able to do it. I was keeping up. I was unable to afford a computer, so I continued to complete my assignments on my trusty and much loved and used electronic typewriter. It took longer to complete work this way compared with the speed of a computer, so, when possible, I would use Uncle Fred and Aunty Bron's computer. I met most of my deadlines and if I was unwell, lecturers were generally supportive in awarding an extension of time.

I was also wonderfully supported by the Student Disability Officer at Deakin. Her name was Margaret McKeough and she helped to make life at uni achievable for me. She ensured that for each semester when I had new lecturers and tutorial teachers, they were aware of my special needs. When it came to exam time, I was able to complete my exams in a special room with other students with disabilities. It was a safe place where I felt I could be myself and be given the time I needed to complete my exams to the best of my ability. Knowing that she was there to support me and my special needs was very comforting.

With each semester of new subjects that came my way, I found most of the content to be manageable. My ability to fully comprehend what I was learning felt great and gave me more confidence. I sought help from lecturers and tutors when I needed it and continued to work to the best of my abilities. I completed every single task from note taking to researching assignments, with dedication and purpose. I tried very hard to make each day at uni count, even when I wasn't enjoying a particular subject very much. The thought of whinging about it made me feel quite ashamed. I didn't wish to squander the opportunities I was being given in being able to attend uni, so whenever other friends were bemoaning the boredom of uni life, I did not participate but tried to subtly remind them how good it was to even be here.

However, my principled approach to be a gracious uni student was seriously challenged when I began a subject called Food Science. It was basically the study of food chemistry. I had never completed chemistry at school – not even one bit in a general science class, due to missing so much school. I found this subject extremely challenging. Many tears and head held in hands moments! Not being able to fully understand what I was learning rocked my self-confidence and generated a lot of stress and worry for me. The thought of failing made me anxious. If I failed that subject, I would not graduate on time and would have to either repeat the subject or do a different one.

Adding to my feelings of anguish, our lecturer was not helpful at all. She was frosty, short-tempered, impatient and severe. And, very old. Simply, not approachable (I promise I'm not be ageist here!) I was on my own. I remember reading everything over and over, highlighting everything left, right and centre and just doing my best. Thankfully, I scraped through but, gee, it was a close call. Another moment of relief and a realisation that even though I was coping at uni, the true impact of missing out on so much school previously was very real and continued to show its impact on my life.

Along the way, I encountered another challenging subject that focused on nutrition. The lecturer would go so fast that a few of us would place tape recorders down the front on the lecturer's lectern, so we could record every word she said. I would take my recordings and play every single word back and write down each word by hand. It took me hours and probably longer than it should take, as I was challenged by the Raynaud's in my hands. Wow, when I think back to how much work it was, with all modesty, I am even more proud of my achievements. These were the days before the internet, before PowerPoint and slideshows, where research for assignments was completed by combing through books, periodicals and journal articles accessible only at the campus library. A time when emailing your lecturers for help was not available. How different it is now for uni students, many of whom hardly ever attend a lecture, as they can watch them via the internet at home. They can even download their notes and listen to podcasts of lectures. Amazing. (Come to think of it, they don't really have to get out of bed, do they?)

I wonder if this generation realise how amazing these advances in technology truly are. They have grown up in a world where everything is available by just a click of a button. I know for myself, I would have been able to conserve so much more energy if all of these resources were available to me back then. How much time would I have saved by simply downloading a PowerPoint file, instead of rewriting pages and pages of lecture recordings? If I was too unwell to attend a lecture, I could have watched it from home. I have no doubt that other students with disabilities who completed uni at the same time I did would be in awe of how interactive education is these days, that they too would have been able to manage their health and their disability with more ease and support.

The developments of technology and how we use it in our everyday life moves so fast. Too fast I think, and maybe people forget to stop and reflect on how the lives of the sick and disabled have been enhanced by the availability of these resources. Technological advances for life at uni are now enabling sick and disabled students to participate in the world with even more inclusiveness and support. And for that, I am truly grateful, as the world is enriched by their contributions.

Chapter Fifteen

Being Lumped with More Worry

During my third year of uni, February 1996, I found a lump in my right breast. It sat near my rib cage. I remember when I found it, I asked Rebecca to check it, to see if she could feel a lump too. Unfortunately, she did. Being so unwell herself, I didn't want to worry Mum, so I told Dad and asked him to stay quiet until I had it confirmed by my GP. Upon examination by my GP, she found two lumps; the one I had found and another lump in my right breast, positioned much higher, near my armpit. She ordered me to have an ultrasound immediately and instructed me to begin vitamin B therapy. I was to take vitamin B6 and evening primrose oil daily to reduce the lumpiness in my breasts.

I was a little shocked that there were two lumps but felt that, hopefully, it was a good sign – safety in numbers. My GP felt confident that there was nothing sinister there and I was too young, twenty years old, to be at risk for breast cancer, particularly without any history of breast cancer in my family. When I eventually told Mum, she was naturally worried and concerned. Her health wasn't great and I did not wish to add to her worries. But this was the situation I found myself in and I felt it best to let her know what I was experiencing.

I went to have the ultrasound on my own and it proved to be an unnerving experience. The radiologist performed the ultrasound on both breasts. He appeared agitated by the results appearing on the screen and excused himself from the room. He returned with a colleague and then proceeded with the ultrasound all over again for a second opinion. After their initial concerns, they concluded that all appeared fine on the screen. This was confirmed in my follow-up visit to my GP a couple of days later. The lumps did not appear to be cancerous, according to the ultrasounds. She suggested that I complete a six-week course of vitamin B6 and evening primrose oil therapy. If these lumps had not shrunk after four weeks or so, a specialist visit would be organised.

After four weeks, the lumps had not disappeared and I was sent to see a general surgeon. Well, what an experience this proved to be. She was around forty years old and had a very brisk and blunt bedside manner. Upon examining both breasts, she concluded that she couldn't feel any lumps at all and told me that my breasts were simply swollen due to hormonal changes in my menstrual cycle. This blew me away. At this stage, these lumps had been sitting there for over six weeks and possibly much longer. To imply that they were swollen because I had my period was laughable to me. I asked her if these lumps did not disappear, would she be prepared to surgically remove them? Her response was staggering. She said, 'No, because you would only have an unnecessary scar and at your age, well …'

For a doctor, a female one at that, to refuse to surgically remove these two possibly very harmful lumps for reasons of vanity and my youth, I believe, was appalling. Even worse was how she could not clearly detect two lumps that had been present in my breast for some time, which had been confirmed by my GP and via ultrasound by not one, but two radiologists, was astounding. My health and possible survival were the priority here, not how I would look afterwards if I needed surgery. It felt like she had completed a very rushed examination of my breasts and I wondered if it was because she did not think I was a liability for breast cancer at the tender age of twenty. I wasn't sure. She simply told me to continue with the vitamin B therapy and to see her in three months' time for a follow-up appointment.

I did not bother seeing her again. After receiving treatment and advice like that, it felt like I'd be wasting my time. I felt dismissed and ignored. I felt frustrated. I resigned myself to the fact that the only thing I could keep doing was to monitor the presence of these lumps and hope that the vitamin B therapy would successfully shrink both lumps within weeks. The troubling feelings of not having definitive answers for this new health issue were another flashback to the complexities of successfully diagnosing my lupus. More anguish. More grey areas in my life. More limbo. Very familiar territory for me, but in hindsight, proved to be invaluable in this experience, as it gave me the strength I needed for moving through each step of this worrying time.

* * *

Serendipity is an amazing thing. There are moments in life where you stop and think, wow, that was meant to be. Within the darkness of this situation, a light was shone on an extremely fortuitous moment, when I met an amazing nurse on a health promotion placement a month or so later. For a subject I was studying, students were sent out on a placement at a health clinic for a month to observe health care practice in action. My placement was at the Maternal and Child Welfare Clinic in rural Whittlesea, twenty minutes up the road from home. Each week, I attended post-natal clinics for mothers. During one of these weeks, the theme was breast care and self-examination. Specifically, how to detect a breast lump. I couldn't believe it. How timely.

I completed the class with the ladies and learnt how to properly self-examine my breasts. Afterwards, I approached the nurse and asked her if I could seek her advice. I told her about my breast lumps and the medical treatment I had received so far. At this stage, the lump that was near my armpit appeared to have shrunk as I could not feel it at all. Unfortunately, the lump I had first discovered, near my rib cage, was still there, just as distinctive as ever.

When I finished my story, the nurse went silent. She then said simply and firmly, 'If you have loved ones, and you don't want them to be standing over your grave, heartbroken and crying for your loss, you must seek another opinion and have this lump removed.' I shuddered. The harsh truth of her words went straight to my heart and I felt sick. She was absolutely right.

At this stage, it had been two months of dithering around the idea that a bunch of vitamin pills would solve this problem, rather than approaching and treating me with concern and immediacy. This nurse had clarified within a few words, the urgency of finding the solution to treating my breast lump. Her insight into my situation was invaluable. I thanked her so much and reassured her that I would do everything I could to take care of myself.

I returned to my GP and conveyed my frustrations, particularly with the hopeless surgeon she had referred me to. It turned out that there was a female GP at the clinic I attended who specialised in women's health and my GP suggested I see her for another opinion.

When my appointment with her arrived, I told her how frustrated and dissatisfied I had been with my treatment by the medical profession so far. She, too, was quite a confident, brisk woman but she was also compassionate and considerate – qualities definitely missing in the other female surgeon. She, too, concluded that having this lump untreated for so long was of genuine concern. I asked if she knew of a surgeon who could perform a biopsy of my lump. Incidentally, her husband was a surgeon. She reassured me that he could do that for me and that I would have a much more positive experience with him, compared with the female surgeon I had seen previously. Finally. A positive step forward.

The appointment with the male surgeon was a few weeks later. Again, off I went on my own to seek his opinion. Mum was too sick to attend with me and Dad was at work. I was okay. Visiting doctors and the like was, unfortunately, a normal and familiar occurrence for me at this young age. The male surgeon was a quiet-mannered, middle-aged man. He performed a fine-needle biopsy and confirmed the seriousness of the lump, particularly as it had been present, unchanged in size, for a few months now. He suspected I was suffering from a fibroid tumour, which is traditionally full of soft tissue and fluid. These tumours are usually benign and would shrink over time.

Pleasingly, the biopsy results confirmed no traces of cancer, however, that didn't mean that the lump should be left as is. The surgeon advised me to continue taking the vitamin B therapy, with the addition of B1, and said that if the lump had not disappeared within three weeks, he would operate and take it out.

Three weeks passed and still no change to the lump. I visited the surgeon again to inform him, but he changed his mind and advised that I wait another three weeks to see if the lump had shrunk. I was to continue taking the vitamin B therapy. Whilst I felt exasperated, I knew I was in good care with him as a physician, so I watched and waited for possible changes in the lump for another three weeks.

Again, three weeks later and still no change in the size of the lump. So, off I went to the private hospital, which happened to be across the road, and I booked myself in for an excision biopsy, to be performed in another three weeks' time. The lump was finally coming out. Thank goodness. Still more time to wait through but at least I was much closer to having it removed.

On the 18th of June, 1996, I finally had the ghastly lump removed, three and a half weeks shy of my twenty-first birthday and around six months after the lump had been diagnosed. I was in surgery for about an hour and home within a day. The surgeon said that it was a stressful procedure, as it was not the classic fibroid tumour he assumed it was. My lump contained dense, fibrous tissue that was not indicative of a fibroid tumour. He was relieved to conclude that this mysterious lump was not cancerous. In fact, he looked incredibly relieved. And so was I.

I didn't realise how long I had been quietly holding my breath all these months, as I felt my body drop and rest more easily after hearing this good news. Six months is a long time to have a breast lump, with no definitive description of whether it was truly benign or cancerous. I had dodged another bullet. My joy was indescribable and my smile widened once more. I wrote a letter of sincere thanks to the nurse who put me on the path to wellness. She was delighted to hear that the lump was benign and pleased that she could be of help to me during this time. I don't think she will ever truly know just how fortuitous her help really was.

* * *

Throughout this distressing time, I had been very anxious about how the ongoing worry of this breast lump was impacting on my lupus. I was told time after time by my rheumatologist, that I had to reduce stress, at all costs. Well, that was easy for him to say. As I was continuing to learn that, just because I had lupus, this did not automatically eliminate me from further life challenges. And when your heart is burdened with fear and worry like mine was, there was only so much I could do to keep my lupus symptoms under control.

To counteract the effects of the surgery and the experience itself, I was ordered by my rheumatologist to spend a week in bed, no matter how good or bad I felt. I was also given an increase of steroids to help control my lupus. So that's what I did. I popped those pills and I stayed in bed that whole week. With more steroids pumping, I felt better than I thought I would post surgery. It was a worrying time, though, as I had a four-week student teaching placement beginning the following week. I hoped and prayed that my lupus would stay under control so that I could commence my teaching rounds without interruption.

Thankfully, I was strong enough the following week to begin student teaching rounds. I had my breast scar taped and bandaged up each day. I was a little uncomfortable, but I managed to make it through each day of my rounds. It was exhausting but it felt great to be there. I didn't mention my operation to anybody. I didn't mention having lupus. I figured I would speak up and say something to my supervisor if I wasn't feeling well. Until then, I promised myself I would simply enjoy being able to participate, to simply do my best without fuss and continue my love of learning how to be a teacher.

* * *

In revisiting this time in my life, I find six months to be simply an unacceptable length of time for a woman to have to wait to remove a suspicious breast lump. Was it because I was twenty years old? Most likely. This makes me angry. The fact that I was a lupus sufferer as well, makes me angrier. Angrier because my body was (and still is) under siege. My immune system completely weakened and suppressed. For medical professionals to repeatedly say, 'Let's wait a few more weeks', over and over and over, just to see if this lump magically 'disappeared', was a complacent and somewhat ignorant approach in not only addressing the threat of breast cancer, but also, in treating a patient with an incurable autoimmune disease such as lupus.

Yes, each and every doctor I consulted during this time was aware that I had lupus. But did they really know how serious lupus was? Looking back, I am not convinced. Any additional health issues, such as a breast lump, that lupus sufferers have to battle, should be treated swiftly, with immediate action. Trying to manage and reduce the severity of a life-threatening disease in lupus was not treated as a priority by the doctors

I consulted with during this time. Controlling my lupus only became an issue during and after surgery, when the breast lump had been removed. Ideally, managing my lupus should have been front and centre across the whole experience of treating my breast lump as well. Instead, it was an afterthought. Maybe I am to blame for not demanding more attention here. Unfortunately, having a breast tumour brought with it a whole new strain of fear for me to endure. It successfully blocked out the daily threat of lupus for me. Completely.

As mentioned previously, in the thirty years that I have suffered from lupus, I have had to repeatedly educate doctors of its symptoms, causes and treatments. It truly astounds me. Disappointingly, in this present day, I don't feel the medical profession is any more advanced in their awareness of lupus and the seriousness in which it must be treated. There are a select, few doctors I have met who have demonstrated how familiar they are with lupus, but they are a rarity.

I keep asking myself, all of these years later, should I have been more demanding? More insistent that the lump be taken out, no matter what? Maybe. I was so young. Breast cancer was not considered a threat for a twenty-year-old woman like me in 1996. Thankfully, that attitude has been banished, as we now know that all women and men, regardless of age, are a risk for breast cancer and must be life-long, vigilant carers of their breast health to try and prevent the spread of breast cancer.

Having this breast lump at such a tender age, increased my awareness of how vulnerable Lupus Warriors are in developing tumours like this. I have read many stories where Lupus Warriors have been diagnosed with either benign or malignant tumours. Brain tumours are particularly common. Not only as lupus sufferers are we vulnerable to developing tumours because our bodies think our own cells are enemy cells, but the immunosuppressant medications and chemotherapies we undertake on a long-term basis make us a target for cancers such as lymphoma.

However, in the mainstream, people wouldn't be aware of this. Nor would they know, that sufferers of other autoimmune diseases such as rheumatoid arthritis and Crohn's disease, are also at risk. That the very medication being used to treat our symptoms, which is helping to save our lives, can also be the cause of ending it. That we are constantly looking over our shoulder, examining and agonising over any new or strange symptoms, hoping and praying that we do not develop other autoimmune diseases, for which we are already at risk, or develop further complications such as cancers, due to the treatments we must take in order to have the quality of life that we deserve. That must change. The myriad of complex autoimmune diseases, and the impact of long-term immunosuppressant treatments used to treat these diseases, must garner more education and awareness amongst our medical profession. Our GPs and specialists must be on alert whenever these diseases present themselves, particularly in conjunction with the threat of, or worse, the presence of suspect tumours. Our survival depends on it.

Chapter Sixteen

Another Step Forward

Not being well enough to work a part-time job throughout uni, was very difficult for me. I always felt very self-conscious around my uni mates. I wasn't flush with cash like they were and I was unable to share stories with them about life in the workplace. I already felt different because I was ill, but socially, I struggled at times to overcome my feelings of loss at not being able to have the lives they were living.

One day at the beginning of my final year at uni, all of that changed. I was approached by one of my lecturers. She told me of an internship that was offered by one of the most elite private schools in Melbourne. At the beginning of each year, the internship was offered to a student studying to become a Human Development and Food Technology Secondary school teacher. It was the job of my lecturer to select a worthy student. Out of all the students training to be teachers in this field, she selected me as a worthy candidate and offered me the internship.

I was extremely humbled to be chosen. With much thought in regard to managing my lupus, I said yes. I had classes spread out over four days a week and the day I was expected to work would be a Friday. I had enough rest time during the week and over the weekend to hopefully manage this change in my routine. I thought to myself, 'Well, if it works out and I am well enough to cope with the demands of working this day, then great. If not, then I had tried to see what was possible.' Aside from further developing my skills as a teacher, I would be earning my very own money. The possibility of being able to do that for the first time felt wonderful.

The internship felt very much like a 'girl Friday' job. The school was five minutes away from the Rusden Campus, which was handy. It was extremely wealthy and well-resourced. I was a nervous wreck driving through the school gates on my first day. The buildings were huge and intimidating. It felt like I had travelled a few kilometres before I had even parked my car! There was only one Human Development and Food Technology teacher at the Senior Campus of this college, so this teacher needed support. Hence, the position of an internship had been specifically created to assist her in any capacity in which she needed help.

I would arrive at 8 am each Friday morning not knowing what I was expected to do for that day. It could be anything. She could ask me to come up with a short-answer revision test for her Year 12 Human Development class. I would be expected to read the relevant chapters of the text she was using and come up with appropriate questions to challenge her students. Just like that, and it would have to be typed and finished well before the end of the day. I could be asked to spend the day in the school's amazing printing room, printing and binding health workbooks for her Year 10 Health Education classes. I could also be asked to preview educational videos for her and decide which one's were suitable to purchase. Completing her photocopying and a myriad of other organisational tasks would also fill the day.

However, the tasks that would shock me the most were those that I had to complete in the college industrial kitchen. It was the only operational kitchen for students to use at the college, in their VCE Food Technology studies. Only a handful of students had selected Food Technology as a VCE subject, so the space was just big enough to store relevant food materials that were then transported to the classroom kitchens of a neighbouring school, where these students would cook. I was often asked to make sure relevant kitchen equipment and ingredients were ready for student use. Whilst there was no official food assistant to permanently complete these jobs, I was constantly amazed at how spoon-fed these students were. So much preparation was done for them.

The most memorable preparation task I had to complete was organising the transportation of ingredients of a fruit cake to the neighbouring school's kitchen. Instead of organising the collection of tubs of flour, sultanas, fruit peel, etc. for students to access and then measure themselves for their own cakes once they had arrived at the neighbouring school, I was asked to measure out every single ingredient that each student would need to make their cake. I had about six large plastic bags spread out and I would go through each ingredient needed to make the cake, carefully measuring out the correct amount for each student. Effectively, all students had to do was pick up the bag of ingredients, pour them into a bowl and mix them with the addition of a couple of liquid ingredients, and their fruit cake mix would be ready to place into a pre-prepared cake tin, ready to bake.

Simple but completely void of the development of actual cooking skills. These students were about seventeen, even eighteen years old, and they were having their ingredients pre-prepared for them. It was shocking to me, coming from a government school, to see how pampered these students were. It made me angry. Angry, because I couldn't help but think of my experience as a sick student in a public school and how challenging school was for me. Seeing the wealth and privilege available to these students was hard.

Ultimately, I felt sorry for them, because I believed that these students were not being shown a realistic view of the world ahead of them. They were not in an environment that exposed them to more diversity, such as working and socialising with other students with physical or learning disabilities. They were not benefiting from the lessons that adversity brings. The level of academia they were seeing amongst their student cohort was similar to their own. They were not witness to the mixed abilities that would exist within an average public school classroom. When they finished school, they were not going to be pampered throughout uni or in their workplace. They were going to be treated like everyone else, so this false sense of entitlement was going to be short-lived and their resilience truly tested once they were outside these school walls.

I would complete tasks like these with much diligence, but it made me reflect on what type of teacher I wanted to be. Seeing this cossetted approach to learning, reinforced my belief that, ideally, students should co-exist in an educational setting where equality and opportunity for all, regardless of ability, was the focus. An inclusive environment where diversity and individuality are celebrated, and student performance is achieved on their own merits. I realised that my values on education were not aligned with those I was seeing in this elitist private school setting. A teaching environment like this was not for me.

Not only was I gaining an insight to how exclusive, elite private schools operated, I was also gaining an insight into how it felt to be treated as a non-teaching member of staff in a workplace like this. Over time, I felt like I was treated as a 'nobody'. I would show up every Friday in the offices where I worked, for a whole year, and hardly any of the teachers acknowledged me. Barely anyone asked my name or was even remotely interested in my position at the school. There was a small staffroom near the office; plenty of room and space for other teachers to sit down and chat (It was actually awesome. A couple of stories high with beautiful garden views, cosy couches and chairs, unlimited tea and coffee and assorted cream biscuits available all the time. Assorted creams!). As lovely as it was to take a break, I actually dreaded it, as I did not look forward to the feeling of being overlooked and ignored by these teachers. I would sit with the office ladies, which was nice, but the segregation amongst staff felt awful. A true hierarchy existed, with teachers at the top and non-teaching staff beneath them.

At the end of the year when my job came to a close, I wasn't given a proper farewell by the school administration. In fact, I wasn't formally thanked or farewelled at all. I sat at the farewell function and waited to be acknowledged and thanked by the teacher I had been working for. Nothing. Absolutely nothing. It felt awful, sitting there and watching one staff member after another, being valued and recognised for their efforts, whilst it seemed that I had not been deemed worthy enough to be acknowledged for the small contribution I had made to their school community throughout the year. Whilst I was so grateful for the opportunity to further develop my teaching skills, I was relieved when the year was over.

* * *

In regard to managing my lupus during my last year of uni, with working one day a week, I coped reasonably well. I rarely missed a Friday of working, but at times, it was a challenge. I felt the weight of remaining in good health. I was always terrified of having a lupus flare, and worse, terrified of revealing to my employer how sick I really was. I didn't mention that I had lupus to the teacher I worked with. I simply hoped and prayed that I was able to hold on and be able to sustain working one day a week.

I was scared of sharing that I had lupus. I was afraid of being ostracised or discriminated against. This was my first real job in the workplace and I was truly terrified of being shown the door if my lupus flared. I had experienced ignorance in my young life and was wise enough to know that not everybody responded with concern or kindness when they learned that I was ill. Having lupus made it even harder, because hardly anyone even knew what lupus was back then (and still don't today). The fact that I was able to attend uni and look seemingly well by appearance, made it even more challenging to convey to people how seriously ill I was. Even though I was whippet thin with a puffy, bloated face, I was a smiling, cheery person. Convincing others that I was struggling with my health was fraught with judgement. It was easier to keep quiet and keep my head down.

Life experiences had also taught me to be apprehensive about revealing my illness, as I was scared about the reaction I would receive. Would it be one of genuine concern? Or would it be a dismissive reaction, with people not wishing to know more or understand how lupus was affecting me? I always felt conflicted. In my heart, I did not feel ashamed that I had lupus and I wanted to be more forthcoming, but my shyness in discussing my personal life continued to challenge me. Additionally, to have experienced cruel reactions to my illness by members of my own family, I was trying to protect myself from experiencing anymore hurt. Despite the love and support I received from my immediate family, consciously or unconsciously, my aunty and granny had taught me, to some extent, to feel shame for being ill. So, in many ways, I was always trying to be my own protector.

Ultimately, I figured that if I became ill and was unable to work for a period of time or even continue working, then I would then have to be forthcoming and reveal that I had lupus, whatever the consequences. But if I was able to manage my role as an intern, then I would keep my lupus struggle to myself. Reducing unnecessary stress is integral in trying to prevent lupus flares. I was trying to pick my battles and reduce unnecessary lupus flares. I just wanted to be well.

LUPUS = *Lift Up, Persevere, Use Strength*

* * *

Even though I was being secretive in my workplace about having lupus, toward the end of my degree, I attended a conference that focused on students with disabilities and it opened my mind. All the students at Deakin Uni with disabilities were invited to spend the day together with a range of professors and lecturers from the uni to discuss the challenges we had as students with a disability whilst studying at uni. It was such an interesting, enlightening day. Students in attendance represented a wide range of disabilities from permanent injuries and paraplegia, to intellectual disabilities such as autism and chronic illnesses, like mine.

We were asked during the day to write a short piece explaining how it felt to have a disability at uni. Some of us offered to read our stories (not me, of course!) to give the lecturers a greater insight and understanding of how we felt as students with special needs. I was really moved by the stories shared. These students had similar fears, anxieties and insecurities as I did. They worried about whether they would make it through uni to achieve their degrees, of how that would then transpire into a sustainable career. Would they be seen as talented workers with much to offer? Or would they be 'passed over', their disability possibly slighting the opinions of those in charge of deciding their fate in the workplace?

I felt as though for the first time I was surrounded by like-minded people. It was pivotal in the process I was making my way through, feeling more comfortable and at ease saying out loud that I suffered from lupus. It helped me so much to feel less alone. In many ways, I found it more helpful to learn of the many struggles these students were experiencing than I would have if I was in a room full of fellow lupus sufferers. I was able to develop more empathy and admiration for those students who were struggling with their studies much more than I was. My eyes were opened to pain and suffering in other forms besides lupus. It was very grounding to stop and reflect on my life at that time and to see all of the things I was still able to do. I was independent, able to drive to and from campus, strong enough to concentrate and study for longer periods of time than I thought possible and, best of all, I was succeeding at making each day count. It was not lost on me how great it felt to be at uni and able to work one day a week as an intern. Even though I was being secretive about having lupus in my workplace, meeting these students encouraged me to be less self-conscious and more comfortable talking about my illness.

The stories we wrote, were collected and published in a special edition of a Deakin Uni publication. Not long after attending the conference, I was contacted by a lady named Professor Marjorie Martin. She was a professor of Biology at Deakin and she had read my story in the uni publication. She wanted to meet with me. I was intrigued.

Our meeting was in her office at Deakin Uni's Burwood campus. A middle-aged lady who was very kind in manner, commented on the strength of my writing in the story I had written for the publication. She said that out of all of the stories shared by the students, mine spoke of hope and positivity. I was, and still am, very humbled to hear that my impromptu story, hurriedly and nervously written, had made such an impact. She then told me of her work as a writer of a VCE Biology textbook for VCE students. She and a co-author had written a few editions of this text. In particular, they liked to intersperse each topic they featured by including real-life stories to help students understand how biology exists in real life. For example, a chapter on chromosomes might feature an accompanying case study on twins.

After reading my story about lupus, Professor Martin had the idea that for her chapter on autoimmune diseases, I could write a case study of my experience with lupus. This would hopefully help students understand what autoimmune diseases were, specifically lupus, and to give them an insight into how lupus can affect one's life. I would have a word limit and, if possible, provide her with a photo to also accompany the article and be published in the text. I was very honoured to be sought out in this way, to be offered an opportunity to produce a written piece for a book! I found some courage and said yes.

By the time my case study article was published in the textbook, I had graduated from uni. It was very fitting then, to be able to provide a photo of myself in my cap and gown to accompany my article. When I first opened the textbook and turned the pages to see my story and my photo, I felt very proud and quite emotional. For anyone reading my story who happened to have lupus or knew someone who suffered from lupus or a chronic disease, I was demonstrating that with love, support and faith in myself, I was able to find a way forward and succeed in life. Maybe, they could too.

Adapting to life with lupus was proving to be my biggest teacher, as I had never imagined that I would be comfortable enough to share my suffering and the challenges that I had experienced. It was a little confronting to see my thoughts and feelings out there on the written page for students and teachers to read, but at the same time, I felt as though I had taken another step forward in accepting my life as a chronically ill person. That in some small way, by sharing my story, I was not only making a difference in creating greater awareness of what lupus is, I was providing a voice on behalf of the chronically ill, who are more often than not forgotten and marginalised people.

Chapter Seventeen

Achieving the Unachievable

After the endurance test of making my way through secondary school and four years of intensive study at uni, the end of my final year provided many unexpected, shining moments for me. In every student teaching placement, I felt very at peace with my decision to become a teacher. I loved teaching and watching myself gain more self-confidence and competence within the classroom. I felt reassured that I was following the right path for me. I loved creating and preparing my lesson plans, putting them into practice in the classroom and then reflecting on areas of refinement and improvement in which I needed to keep building. I loved being with the students, particularly those moments when there was time for a laugh. Building a lovely camaraderie with them was showing me that this was the most integral aspect of becoming a successful teacher. If students could see my humanity, that I was friendly, fair but firm and most importantly, forgiving, then mutual respect would be achievable.

I was also learning that students are examining you the whole time you are standing before them; what I am wearing, how I am wearing it, the suitability of my make-up, the sound and tone of my voice, whether I was on time each lesson, how organised I was – even my choice of pencil case and folders, and if I was demonstrating care and dedication in my work for them. If I passed their acceptance test, they were then most likely to respond by working to their potential. Being an encouraging, approachable and caring teacher mattered.

It was such a grounding experience and one where I took much time listening to feedback and advice from my student teacher mentors in each of the school's I worked in during those four years. It was the best way to develop and grow as a student teacher. I am not a fan of the current hurried and varied ways of becoming a teacher. In my experience, some graduate teachers, specifically those who have come from an established career prior to teaching, who are fast-tracked into teaching with reduced teaching degrees, lack the growth, reflection and patience needed to become truly capable and competent in the classroom. I was grateful to have those years to mature and develop my teaching skills at a sensible pace. I was more certain of my abilities, more confident in my approach and in my sense of self.

Amazingly, I had passed all of my subjects during my four years of study. Most of them extremely well. So well, that I was awarded membership of the 'Golden Key National Honour Society', in 1997, in recognition of Outstanding Scholastic Achievement and Excellence. In addition to this amazing achievement, I was honoured with the award for Student of the Year in my teaching field, Home Economics. I shared this exciting honour with another student in my course. We were both awarded this title as we had the highest marks in our course. I honestly couldn't believe it. My goal was to do my very best in being a dedicated student. To persevere and see what I could achieve. I never imagined that I would receive such amazing accolades at the end of my degree. I was overwhelmed with feelings of surprise, joy and, ultimately, pride.

My family felt all of those feelings too. Particularly, my parents. They were so delighted that I had successfully completed uni and had been able to overcome periods of illness during this time to complete my double degree within the four years allocated. They were prepared for possible moments of ill health that may have held me back and delayed the completion of my double degree. It truly was a remarkable feat and an incredibly defining moment and achievement for me. I had proven that anything is possible in life, particularly when one has love, support, positivity and hope on their side. I felt as though achieving this award was a sign – a blessing that I was where I was meant to be in life, that believing in myself and my dream of becoming a teacher was being validated in a most special way.

I received both of these awards in special ceremonies at Deakin Uni. In particular, it was very exciting to hear my name called out when I was given my award for Student Teacher of the Year for Home Economics. I had to walk onto a stage to the sound of applause for my achievement. I was very moved. I just couldn't believe it, and to this day, I reflect on this moment with much pride and affection.

It was equally as thrilling to hear my name called out during my graduation ceremony for my double degree. An incredible moment, one I hoped I would be able to achieve, and to have done just that, was extremely gratifying. I had succeeded. I had become a secondary school teacher. For all of those people who had doubted me, knocked me, criticised me; well, it didn't stop me. And I'm so glad. For I would not have had the enriched, rewarding career I have had in my life in being a teacher. The privilege of trying to make a difference in the lives of my students. And for many of those doubters, they missed out on seeing the highs and lows I had experienced in order to achieve my dream. It would be their loss, for they had missed out on seeing a Lupus Warrior in action.

Part Three

Use Strength

Living with Hope and Perspective

Chapter Eighteen

The Art of Disclosure

How do I integrate myself within the watchful, judging eye of the workplace? How do I suffer without complaint, without subjecting myself to the possibility of prejudice? Do I reveal that I have lupus? If so, how much do I disclose? Does it mean that I haven't accepted my fate, that yes, I am diseased, if I keep it hidden from others? Or am I being smart, wise even, to protect myself from being subjected to further hurtful, insensitive comments from ignorant people in the world?

When I first began teaching, I still wasn't sure how to approach the topic of having lupus with a prospective employer. It's not something to blurt out in the middle of a job interview, is it? When I was successful in being employed as a teacher for the first time, I was twenty-two years old and had been appointed a six-month, full-time contract based on my own merits. When I began teaching at this particular school, I was both excited and terrified in equal measure. Excited because I had an opportunity to teach, on my own, for the very first time and to put into practise lots of ideas I had buzzing around in my head. Terrified, because I was so young and teaching on my own for the first time. I would be just four years older than my students in my Year 12 Human Development class! I was also terrified of becoming ill, of having a lupus flare and missing significant periods of time from school.

My workload was very confronting. The faculty I had joined was disorganised and they had not developed current teaching resources to match curriculum standards. It was up to me to devise my own teaching plans, based on Junior, Middle and Senior School teaching requirements. It was an incredibly demanding workload for a graduate, let alone a chronically ill graduate like me. I was given five Year 7 Food Technology classes, one Year 9 Food Technology Class, one Year 11 VCE Human Development class and one Year 12 Human Development class. This teaching allotment was huge! In the late nineties, if you were deemed qualified to teach, then you taught whatever was given to you – unlike today's expectations of graduate teachers in Victoria's State Education system, where reduced teaching loads and appointed teaching mentors are the norm.

Over time, certain situations would arise where I was confronted with having to explain that I had lupus. More so with the teachers in my faculty. Lupus would arise in conversation after a time because when I was frequently asked what my plans were for the weekend, I was very low key about them. 'Just taking it easy' as my go to response started to wear thin, for I was a seemingly young, vibrant twenty-two-year-old and, in the eyes of my peers, I should be out living it up and socialising every weekend. They would look at me a little suspiciously. After a while, I explained that I had a condition called lupus. Unsurprisingly, no one knew what that was. However, it was a relief to share this. Another small step forward in being more comfortable coming out of my shell and divulging more about myself. It also meant that if I was struggling, hopefully my colleagues would be supportive and understanding. It was a risk I was learning that I had to take, regardless of the outcome. It was becoming clearer to me that hiding behind lupus was simply futile.

Working in a school environment meant that aside from working with teaching colleagues in my faculty, I was also liaising and working with a range of teachers from other subject areas. Whilst having divulged my lupus to members of my faculty during my first teaching job, other facets of my teaching role such as yard duty requirements became an issue, where having lupus was not going to be something I could keep quiet.

I remember being allocated my first yard duty responsibilities. All of them required me to be outside in open, sun-filled spaces. I didn't know what to do. My doctors had instructed me not to be in the direct rays of the sun. Walking outside from one side of the school to the other was fine as I was moving and not in a position where the UV rays would be penetrating for very long. But standing for twenty to twenty-five minutes outside in direct contact with the sun was banned, for I could develop a full-blown lupus flare due to the intensity of the UV ray exposure.

I didn't know what to do because getting a teaching job in the late nineties was extremely hard, let alone getting a permanent one. Whilst my first teaching job was a definitive six-month contract with no possibility for permanency, I was anxious not to be seen as 'difficult'. My performance in this job was crucial, as I needed to be the most cooperative, dedicated teacher I could be to hopefully gain enough support and recommendation in successfully gaining employment for my next teaching position.

I endured those yard duty placements. I would put my sunscreen and hat on and walked tentatively, scouring for possies out of the sun. I would find undercover shelter and stand under huge, shady trees that would allow me to still fulfil my student supervision role. However, I would feel ashamed of myself. I was ashamed because I knew I should have spoken up and asked the teacher in charge of yard duty allotments to find a more suitable, sun-free spot for me to complete my yard duty. Looking back now, I feel sorry for the twenty-two-year-old me, so frightened to make a fuss, all in the name of wanting to be seen as 'agreeable' and 'employable'.

Yard duty was not the only issue that created a lupus conundrum. Participating in school excursions such as athletics and swimming carnivals and camps, proved to be hurdles as well. Again, it was imperative to my future employment prospects that I be seen as a teacher who was willing to put her hand up and participate in extra-curricular activities. Attending athletics and swimming carnivals was compulsory for all staff. Thankfully, all of the top jobs for these occasions, which were in the blaze of the hot sun, such as supervising the running races, were delegated to the more permanent, experienced and popular members of staff. As a wee graduate and the lowest on the pecking order, I was given the less glamourous jobs, such as canteen supervision or yard duty outside of the toilets. This, thankfully, allowed me to find a position out of the sun.

Again, I didn't put my hand up for support. I didn't seek out the teacher in charge of organising these carnivals to ask for a guaranteed role that allowed me to be out of the sun. These carnivals were long, tiring days for the healthiest of teachers. For me, it meant crashing into bed until I had to get ready for school the next day. I felt exhausted, angry and frustrated at myself for continuing to compromise my health.

* * *

The Year 7 camp in all secondary schools is an important opportunity for the students to socialise and get to know one another in their new school environment. These camps are demanding. So many activities are crammed in over a couple of days. Again, as a graduate teacher, I was encouraged to attend this camp, my first as a qualified teacher for I was seen as a young, energetic teacher – the perfect candidate for a camp of this size. Anxious about being well enough to sustain the level of energy needed in attending this camp, I again kept my lupus to myself and participated in all of the outdoor activities I was given – outdoor swimming in the creek, flying fox and long walks. I would be outside in the sun much longer than I should have been. I knew the risks but still went ahead, putting my job ahead of my health. How foolish I was.

To manage my fatigue, whenever I had a break, instead of having a cuppa and chatting with other teachers, I would quietly sneak off and have a nap. When I returned home from this camp, I was borderline flaring. Full blown lupus butterfly rash, fever, headaches and extreme fatigue. I put myself to bed for a couple of days and then back to school.

Looking back, I was such a scared girl. So, so scared that I wouldn't be recommended for a permanent teaching job if I didn't say yes to what was asked of me. As a new staff member, I didn't know the principal team well enough to trust that I had their understanding and support. I found the prospect of having to explain what lupus was extremely daunting, as I was putting myself in a position to be scrutinised and judged. I didn't want to give an employer a reason not to hire me, for I was sick compared with the healthier candidate. I feared that they could always find other reasons to justify not selecting me, which had nothing to do with me having lupus. Maybe they would point out my unreliability if I was absent too much. Or maybe they would find fault in some aspect of my teaching as a reason not to hire me. They had all of the power. They could do anything.

The Art of Disclosure

* * *

After my six-month contract ended, I was successful in finding another teaching position. I approached this job with the same attitude; I did everything I could to present myself as a viable, healthy, hard-working teacher. This position was actually very suitable for managing my lupus. It was a part-time position, for another six months. I only had to teach three days a week. This was extremely helpful in reducing flares as I could rest on alternate days off. Once again, lupus never came up in the conversation with the principal team and I did my best to present myself as a worthy, employable teacher.

For my third teaching job in less than two years, I continued my approach to discussing lupus in the same way. I confided with the teachers in my faculty area who I was working directly with. With this position, there was a strong possibility that it could become a permanent job to apply for at the end of that year. It was a full-time job and similar to my first teaching position, demanding a huge effort from me. I had been allocated three separate VCE classes. This meant that I had three individual sets of preparation at a senior level; one Year 12 and two Year 11 classes. That, on its own, is another huge workload. Adding to these demands, I also had middle and junior Food Technology classes.

I pushed the fear of lupus flares out of my mind and said to myself, 'I will worry about it if and when a flare presents itself.' Again, I attended camps, sports carnivals, excursions, late night student exhibitions, school plays, etc. My weekend activities were sleeping and marking and planning lessons. Each week, on repeat. But I was struggling. Seriously, just holding on and pushing through increased joint and muscle pain, fevers and headaches. And then, I could push no more.

A flare that lasted a couple of weeks arrived and I had to disclose how much I was struggling. Lupus was winning. But then, it was always going to be the winner. I had to give in and put my faith in humanity, in the hope that people who I disclosed my lupus to, could be trusted and would not be judgemental or use it as a reason not to employ me full-time.

I needn't have worried. When I returned to school after my flare, word had spread amongst some members of staff that I was battling ill health. A teacher who I did not know very well, but who had always been warm and friendly to me in passing, approached me. She offered me a copy of her teaching timetable. She highlighted the periods where she wasn't teaching, her 'spares', and insisted that whenever I was feeling unwell and needed to rest, to come and find her, for she would come and replace me in my classroom. I remember my eyes brimming with tears. I was so overwhelmed by her kindness and thoughtfulness. No one had ever shown me such compassion in the workplace. She felt compelled to offer her support, whenever I needed it. It blew me away.

This one act of kindness was a significant moment for me. It changed how I approached divulging my lupus. I became braver. I found more courage and I started to let go of any self-consciousness I had about sharing that I had lupus. That meant my shyness and quiet nature were stretched and challenged, but in the best way possible.

The step I had taken in sharing my lupus struggle, opened up more moments of kindness and compassion. I suffered another lupus flare not long after this one. Not only did more of the staff know that I had lupus, everyone in my teaching office knew. The office I worked in was made up of art, science and math teachers and it was a lively work space, full of laughter. When I returned to school after a two-week absence, I was given an extra. An 'extra' is assigned to teaching staff to cover for other teaching staff when they are absent from school. Teachers are given these 'extras' if they have a spare period in their teaching load. It means that you lose time that day to complete your marking, lesson prep and the myriad of other administrative tasks that need to be done.

I remember feeling a little shocked to be given an extra on my first day back after two weeks off. I had so much work to catch up on, particularly assessing where students were up to and how they had behaved when I was absent. I only had one spare period that day and now it was gone. I mentioned to a few people in my office that I had an extra. They too, were surprised and thought that was a bit rough, given that I had been absent for so long and needed to ease back into my teaching routine. As annoying as it was, I didn't wish to complain. I had returned to work and was fit for duty, so I had to cop it on the chin!

Unbeknownst to me, one of the science teachers in my office was so upset that I had been given this extra, that he marched down to the daily organiser's office and demanded that this extra was taken off my teaching load for the day and given to someone else. He told the daily organiser that it was unacceptable to expect a teacher coming back from sick leave, to take on additional duties on their first day back. Affronted by his outburst, the suddenly apologetic daily organiser withdrew my extra and gave it to another teacher. I was so relieved. And again, so overwhelmed that another teacher, a colleague, had stood up for me in this way. This act of unfairness was felt by not only me, but by other work colleagues. I felt even more cared for in the workplace and I started to feel less anxious about disclosing that I had lupus.

The goodwill that was evolving as a result of me becoming more comfortable in discussing my ill health then enabled me to help others. When learning of my lupus, another teaching staff member, who later became my dear friend, Maree, approached me with a delicate issue involving a Year 7 student. He had been diagnosed with Type 1 Diabetes and was struggling socially with his peers in regard to sharing his condition. She asked me if I would like to meet up with him and share my story of having lupus with him, in the hope that having another person with an illness to talk to would help him to feel less alone with his experience.

It was one of the most rewarding moments of my teaching career. Being able to share the awkwardness and difficulties of being different, of being sick when you are at school, with this young boy, proved to be helpful for both him and me. It was a moving example of how being vulnerable can cultivate bravery, for with more understanding from others, comes greater self-acceptance and less shame, as he and I were both able to move forward with greater confidence and resolve.

At the end of my first year at this school, I was awarded a permanent position. I didn't even have to be re-interviewed. I had achieved this position on my own merit. It was a wonderful feeling.

* * *

When reflecting on these earlier years of my teaching career, I am moved by the additional angst I felt as a young teacher. I was already under enormous pressure and expectation as a graduate teacher, but I was also contending with so many possible what-if scenarios in my head that related to being judged for having lupus. In retrospect, is it really any wonder, for members of my own family, such as my aunty and grandma, had treated me so cruelly when I was diagnosed with lupus. They saw no hope for me, no potential for me to still find a way to make a difference in this world. They created fear in my heart that not everyone was going to be kind when learning of my plight. Being shy, quiet and sensitive only magnified my need to protect myself from further hurt and disappointment from the world.

But I know I am not alone in feeling this way. Judgement from others is a reality that we as sufferers of chronic, incurable, autoimmune diseases such as lupus fear the most. We are scared of the possibility of being discriminated against, for we don't always look ill. We are not bandaged up or missing limbs; there are often no major visual clues to indicate that we are ill. However, if you do stop and look at us as Lupus Warriors more closely, you may see how bloated our faces are as a result of taking steroids. Or you might see a blotchy, red, raised rash covering our cheeks. We are likely to look a little pale and tired. We worry that not everyone completely understands just how ill we really are. Unbeknownst to many, we are so highly medicated, often on the most toxic drugs you can take, that allow so many of us to be well enough to have the strength and energy to work. Without this medication, we would be extremely ill, bedridden, with a poor prognosis for survival.

I am often asking myself, how do I convince others that my pain is real? That yes, my wide smile is genuine, despite any pain or discomfort I'm feeling. It's one of sheer joy because I am participating in the world. That even though I have lupus, with the assistance of medicine and a positive, determined attitude, I am able to contribute to society and somehow make a difference. It's not always easy in moments when you are sharing your lupus symptoms and are explaining the treatment required to treat them, and some people say, 'Oh, but you look so well' or 'Gee, you wouldn't know it to look at ya.' It feels as though some people who say things like this are not truly listening to me. Maybe they are too busy deciding if I really am ill or not, based on how I look. It has also been my experience that when I have been competent and successful in my career, it can make their assessment of how genuinely ill I am even worse. In moments like this, I can sense the scepticism ticking over in their minds and hear the shift in the tone of their voices as they appraise my achievements. I can see them wondering, 'If you are so ill, how is it that you are happy and good at your job?'

In those moments, I have felt so judged. You can't help but think, 'Am I not allowed to look well and be working regularly, even though I am seriously ill?' Why can't people just say, 'It's wonderful to see you doing well.' Or if you have been unwell and return to work, simply say, 'It's good to see you. How are you?', and just listen to the answer, without comment.

The Art of Disclosure

It's very difficult, as everyone has their own experience of illness or of what they think illness is and looks like. For many people, maybe they have had very limited experience with seriously ill people, which could explain why they are often the ones who are the most ignorant or insensitive with their comments. Over the years, I have experienced a myriad of comments, as many chronically ill people do, particularly when I have returned to work after a lupus flare. I would often be asked, 'What did you do to cause this flare?' I always feel very confronted when asked this question. I find it rude, as it feels as though that person is implying that I have been somehow irresponsible in taking care of my health and that it is my own fault for having a flare. As shared previously, my standard response is, 'Well, no matter how well I manage to take care of myself, I have an incurable disease. It gets to do what it wants, when it wants.' That usually makes them stop and think. Or, at least I hope it does.

When returning to work after extended sick leave, one colleague would always say to me, 'Should you be here?' Again, I would find that question rude and judgemental – another person implying that I wasn't taking care of my health. I would also find this question upsetting, as it meant that I was being judged for my ability to appraise my own symptoms and assess when I was well enough to return to work. To imply that I did not know when I was improving, feeling better and ready to step back into work was upsetting. I would also be offended at this line of questioning, particularly as this person knew I had been battling lupus for many years. I felt like I was being spoken to as if I was a child – someone who didn't know how to take care of herself. The fact that after thirty years of having lupus and I was extremely well informed with lupus symptoms and more than capable of determining when I am feeling better and ready for work, was not acknowledged or respected at all by this person, disappointed me greatly.

But with more thought, I would think, well, this person just doesn't understand. And because this was a comment I received repeatedly when I returned to work after a flare, it meant that it was likely that this person was never going to understand. I had to learn to be a duck and let that water run off my back. For I knew how much I was trying to manage my disease and take good care of myself. I knew my own truth. And that was all that mattered.

I know from my experience, my doctors have always advised me to keep my illness as quiet as I can, which in many ways, has also made it difficult for me to be more comfortable sharing my illness. But this advice comes from a place of compassion, as my doctors have seen the worst of humanity in watching how some of their patients have been treated in the workplace. A story shared with me by my current rheumatologist always brings tears to my eyes. Her patient suffers from ankylosing spondylitis, an inflammatory disease, and works as a secondary school teacher at a private school. The pain she endures requires her to sit down when needed. Despite repeated medical certificates from my rheumatologist requesting that she be able to complete yard duty at a post that would allow her to sit down when she needed to, the school administration disregarded my rheumatologist's medical certificate and insisted that this teacher perform the yard duty posting that she had been assigned; one where she was unable to sit down.

Her experience is distressing to me. The prejudice and lack of compassion shown not only to her as a person, but as a member of their school community, was disgraceful. What amazes me is that she was not looking for a way out of completing her yard duty responsibilities; quite the opposite. She wished to perform her job in the best capacity suitable for her. That her request was ignored, demonstrates just how ignorant and cruel the workplace can be. It perpetuates the hesitance that we as chronically ill people feel about disclosing our illnesses to our employers. Treatment like this, systemically suppresses our voices, which in turn reduces greater awareness in the world of the prevalence of diseases such as lupus and ankylosing spondylitis. Little did I know that I would one day, too, experience my own moments of discrimination in the workplace.

***

Eight years into my teaching career, one employer, the principal of the school, was particularly ruthless in trying to deem me as being in good health and not worthy of being given extended sick leave by the Department of Education. It seemed that if he could prove that I was in good health, he didn't have to retain me as a permanent member of his staff. He knew that I did not wish to return to work at his school. In simple terms, he was trying to get rid of me. I was on sick leave at this stage for about a year, mostly due to extremely exacerbated lupus as a result of a bullying culture in the faculty of this particular school where I worked.

I found myself in a similar situation to the lady with ankylosing spondylitis. The principal, too, refuted and disregarded all medical certificates provided to him from my medical team of doctors that clearly explained how seriously ill I was with lupus. My rheumatologist is one of the best in Melbourne, and to dispel her medical opinion in this way was shocking. (After leaving the care of the Royal Children's Hospital, I regularly visited my first adult rheumatologist that I was referred to. During my appointments, I would often leave his office in tears. I was made to feel bad that I was not strong enough to complete the myriad of exercise regimes the rheumatologist insisted I practice. No one should ever leave a doctor's office like that, especially when you are chronically ill. After around ten years of seeing other rheumatologists, I eventually found a brilliant rheumatologist – compassionate and understanding with a warm, generous personality.) It was extremely distressing to feel disregarded in this way. What was equally devastating about this situation was that my employer had failed to provide a safe work environment for me as a member of his staff, and that I had become extremely ill as a result.

He insisted that I see an independent physician who was employed by the Department of Education to assess, when required, the health status of teachers on sick leave in the State Government system. His job was to physically examine me, assess my medical history and determine if I had lupus. Basically, he was assessing whether or not I was faking my ill health. I had pathology tests that proved I had lupus, years and years of doctor's reports that proved this, but no, this was not good enough for my employer. The distress of having a prospective examination from a complete stranger and the added stress of what it was going to do to my health was not considered at all. But I went through with it. Again, I didn't want a paper trail that made me look like a difficult employee. I desperately needed to get out of this school and I needed my next employer to see me as competent and compliant.

Thankfully, the physician agreed that I was legitimately suffering from lupus. My principal had failed to remove me as a permanent staff member. He just had to wait until I was well enough to return to teaching at another school, in order for me to be given a transfer to have me off his books permanently.

Hearing stories like the yard duty issue experienced by the lady with ankylosing spondylitis, and even the prejudice seen in my own experiences, still makes me very wary of discussing my lupus. But in many ways, it can be seen as a blessing. Enlightening even. For if people are going to be ignorant, mean and cruel, I do not wish to work for or with them. I am so grateful for the acts of kindness that were shown to me during my early years as a teacher, as they paved the way for me to open my heart more widely, with less fear. They showed me it was possible to work in a safe, supportive environment. When I have commenced a new teaching job, I don't immediately mention that I have lupus. But I approach the principal not long after I have started working and share my illness. I reassure them that I am able to perform my teaching duties but that I will have a few special needs. I have become extremely comfortable doing this and have been for many, many years now.

I have also found the courage to introduce myself to the relevant staff members in charge of sporting carnivals so that I can seek support in being able to participate on the day in a reduced capacity or in an area that is out of the sun. I don't put my hand up to go on camps or volunteer for additional school activities. I recognise that camps in particular are just too much for me. I have accepted this. I am not worried about what other teachers think of me for not participating in extra duties. I don't need their approval. I know that I am trying my hardest to be the best teacher I can be for my students – that is all that matters. I don't need to punish myself and risk further illness in the name of proving that I am a worthy, dedicated teacher. I try and demonstrate these qualities in my teaching practice and hope and pray that that is enough. Well, it just has to be, doesn't it?

***

Despite having more insight, I still have a way to go in another area. For I am a VCE Health and Human Development teacher. I have been for nearly twenty years now. I have educated adolescents on the significance of health promotion and the prevention of lifestyle diseases. I have taught them the importance of nurturing their social, mental and physical health in the pursuit of achieving, where possible, optimal health. I have taught them to be true to themselves, to pursue what interests them, to take pride in themselves and to always give their best. I have shared stories of human hardship with them, whether it be those in extreme poverty in developing countries or someone suffering from a chronic illness. I have implored them to be more mindful, aware and empathetic toward the struggles of others. I have encouraged them to be accepting of their own struggles with the knowledge that in life, we all experience challenges but in different shapes and forms.

Yet I am the complete antithesis of this approach in sharing my own health issues, for I have never divulged my own lupus battle to my students. For after all of these years of teaching, despite being reasonably well supported by my employers, I still live in fear. Fear of parents complaining to the school administration for any prolonged absences I may experience due to a lupus flare and how that may have affected the academic progress of their children. Fear of losing my job due to such complaints. Fear of possible discrimination and prejudice. I have struggled with this irony, that I have not always practiced what I preached to my students.

One of the main reasons I have never divulged my lupus diagnosis with my students, is to reduce worry. I have never wanted my students to worry about me. So many of them endure their own worries at home. Coming to school is respite from those troubles. To know that their teacher is struggling only compounds those sorts of stresses, and I don't wish that on them. And I am a private person. My personal life is completely off limits. I don't discuss my romantic life or even share my birthday. I draw that line very clearly. I don't need that level of gratification, or to be popular with my students – receiving their respect has been my priority. I have worked with so many teachers who share so much of themselves with their students, to the point that the line is too blurred; where students know that nothing is off limits. But that doesn't stop me from sharing my life stories with them in other ways that don't compromise my wish to remain private.

When I shared my lupus story in the Biology textbook all those years ago, strangely, I wasn't too worried if senior students in my classes would become aware of my struggles and approach me about it. Not every school used that Biology book, so the odds were low. However, a few years into teaching, I did have a student approach me and compliment me on my story he had read in his Biology text. I was very touched that he felt comfortable enough to speak to me about it as I wasn't one of his teachers and, even more so, because he was kind. I just wish I knew how to be more forthcoming and at peace with sharing my condition with my own students. Writing this book is a good place to start.

Having lupus challenges my endeavour to always be true to myself. It always will. Just when I think I have mastered another step forward in managing my illness, something will come along to test me and give me more pause for reflection in how I am continuing to adapt to life with lupus. And in doing that, I must always continue to rise up, greet that challenge and try harder to stand with my truth – without fear.

Chapter Nineteen

Bully for Me

Having worked as a secondary teacher for nearly 20 years now, I can honestly say that one of the most challenging aspects of managing my lupus has been the relentless, combative strength demanded of me from working with aggressive teaching colleagues that bullied me. The daily rigour of teaching adolescents has been challenging enough, but I have often felt more solace and safety in my classroom, compared with my teaching staffroom. The politics of teaching in the education system would surprise many. Teaching can be brutal. Exhausting. And unforgiving. But it's the petty jealousy and feelings of being threatened by the success and popularity of other teachers that has time and time again continued to shock and disappoint me.

As you know, it has been my dream to be a teacher. To have fulfilled that dream is a gift, considering my lupus diagnosis and the ongoing effort it has taken me to be a productive, effective and reliable teacher. I have always endeavoured to arrive to school each day, punctual and prepared, hoping to do my best and not to be of harm to others. To be an approachable, fair, supportive and dedicated teacher to my students and my colleagues. I've tried hard to never become complacent or too comfortable in my surroundings. Regardless of the school I have worked at, or whether I was happy or unhappy in that teaching environment, I have always tried to rise above any challenges and be as professional, respectful and as kind as possible during each and every working day. My smile continued to be genuine, no matter the distress I was experiencing, for I have been so grateful to be well enough to teach, to work, earn an income and take care of myself financially. My working hours have decreased over the years as my health has deteriorated, but it truly has been such a triumph, as so many Lupus Warriors are unable to work for long periods of time or work at all.

But when I reflect on my teaching career, I have been absolutely appalled by the immaturity and behaviour of some of my teaching colleagues. Unfortunately, it has marred some happy memories of my teaching career. I never envisaged a working environment that would be repeatedly hostile and at times toxic. The roles of the Health and Human Development and Food Technology teachers are predominantly filled by women. All of the faculties I have worked in have been comprised solely of women. A tiny teaching area compared with subjects such as English and Mathematics, they are likely to be very small faculties, often with only two to three teachers.

A small number of women in a small working space has, unfortunately for me, often meant a bullying culture to work within. Instead of women working closely together, supporting one another and nurturing each other's strengths, it has been for the most part the exact opposite experience for me. A combination of either strong, aggressive personalities or passive aggressive personalities – smiling assassins ready to strike when you are not looking. The kind of people that wake up each day ready for a confrontation and looking for a fight; a way to release all of their own insecurities and pent-up bitterness. Quick to lie and to undermine. Easily jealous and resentful. Threatened by the success, popularity and even happiness of others.

I have worked with women who have mentored me in my development as a teacher, encouraging and supporting me with their friendship and time. But as my self-confidence and competence grew, when I began to truly fly on my own as a teacher, they became resentful and often vindictive, for I had come into my own. I had become successful. In all modesty, well liked and highly regarded by staff and students. And that became unacceptable for these women. All would run well in the workplace while I kept my head down, did my work and stayed under the radar. But when my students achieved excellence, the kind that was exceptional, award-winning and worthy of notoriety, I became a target for sniping, undermining and resentment.

I have worked with women who can be seemingly warm, affable and cooperative. Popular amongst staff and students. But if something changed and they didn't get what they want, their selfishness rose to the fore. Unapologetic and defiant, they showed no shame in being hurtful to others, specifically me, in making sure that they always got what they wanted, no matter the harm they caused. For a new day was always coming and this would be their opportunity to reform, revert back to their regular selves and behave as though nothing had happened. A roller-coaster environment to work in, really. For when everything was up and they were happy, that meant my colleagues and I were happy. But when that dip came out of the blue and the roller coaster hurtled to the bottom, these women would bring everyone down with them. You never knew what each day would bring. Walking on eggshells is such an overused phrase but such an apt one when you are trying to describe working with moody women like these, who swing from smiles to vile in mere seconds.

Unfortunately, I was bullied in the workplace in one particular school. It was two against one and so safety in numbers was not on my side. I had no chance, particularly as I was the new team member. Bullying can sneak up on you very quietly, particularly when the bully is someone who has shown you kindness and affection. Both of these women had. I was picked on for being diligent, for being thorough – for being me. No matter how strong I was in standing up to them, no matter how professional and agreeable I endeavoured to be in trying to forgive and make peace with their behaviour, they kept coming for me.

Having lupus made no difference. In some ways, it made it worse. The moment these women finally left me spiritually and physically broken, after three and a half years of relentless bullying and undermining, was when I was experiencing side effects to a strong, toxic medication. I was thirty years old and battling with the treatment of an immunosuppressant medication called methotrexate. An effective cancer drug, it aimed to reduce the inflammation in my body, which would reduce my pain and help keep my lupus under control. Steroids, antimalarials and anti-inflammatories weren't enough anymore. My GP would inject this medicine into me once a week. The first 6 months are the most challenging as your body adapts to this new drug, which also doubles as both poison and life saver. I would often have chronic nausea prior to and after each dose. Intense headaches and fatigue would also arrive. So, there were a few days each week that were extra challenging for me. I kept it quiet and did my best to work through it.

There was one particular week where I was really struggling. I was able to get my work done but slowly. I needed some support and understanding. My colleague knew that I had lupus and I had opened up and explained that I was having methotrexate treatment. Not long after informing her of my struggle, I was late meeting a faculty deadline for her and so I asked for an extension. I explained to my colleague that I wasn't feeling very well due to my methotrexate injections. I was suddenly met with one of the most heartless, callous responses I have ever received. I was told that I could not have an extension. In fact, if I was late in meeting a deadline again, she would sit down with me and make me complete the task until it was done, before I was able to leave work for that day.

I remember the exasperation, the shock of hearing her words. Where was her compassion, her heart? This woman was a wife, a mother, a teacher. I just couldn't comprehend it, even though I knew her to be quite passive-aggressive in her treatment of me over the years. I could not grasp her cruelty. I just needed help, and some kindness and understanding would have been much welcome. I tried explaining, again, that I was having a rough time on my methotrexate injections and that I just wanted to go home to bed. The methotrexate I was taking is a mild form of chemo and it was going to knock me around for a little while. I insisted that I would get the work done as soon as I could after that. But disappointingly, it made no difference. None whatsoever. Would it have made a difference if I suffered from a more well-known disease?

Thank goodness I had a few years of work experience under my belt and had been shown much support and compassion for managing my lupus in the workplace earlier in my career. It gave me the strength and insight I needed to see that her response was clearly in the minority. Without respect or compassion, there was no hope for me in forging a career in this working environment. There was never an apology for her behaviour, despite mediation, after I had sought support from the assistant principal, but it wasn't worth the effort. This was the same principal who doubted the legitimacy of my illness and requested the medical examination from the Department of Education. He was simply ineffective and unresponsive in his care and support for me with lupus. My rheumatologist even intervened, demanding that this persecution of me be stopped immediately, as I was getting sicker and sicker. It made no difference. Unfortunately, the bullying not only continued, it intensified. A determinedness by these women to keep tearing strips off me and crushing my spirit.

This was a devastating experience for me. Devasting is a powerful word. I don't use it lightly. I was so desperate to escape this daily torment that I sought help from a friend and former teaching colleague of mine. He had left the school where I had been previously teaching to begin teaching at a brand-new secondary college in a semi-rural town north of Melbourne. I asked him if there was a possible teaching role for me. He kindly arranged for me to meet with the school's principal. He explained to her the distressing situation I was in and before I knew it, I had been offered a job teaching English and Science to Year 7 students, and to be the acting Science Faculty leader at the school, effective immediately, until the end of the year. It was June at the time of my appointment.

The idea was that I would relieve two current teachers at the school, the English and Science teachers, to enable them time to develop more curriculum programmes. I would teach these subjects until the end of the year while the new Food Technology building was being constructed. The building would be ready the following year, where my role was to develop the curriculum for the Food Technology programme and facilitate the organisation of the kitchen operations. It would be a huge position for me – a promotion. An opportunity for me to grow and to be instrumental in the development of Food Technology subjects at this new school.

I had found this new role overwhelming. It felt like an out-of-body experience. Because it was a new school and only Year 7 students were present, many of the few teachers employed, were teaching well outside their trained and preferred teaching areas. I was in charge of a Science Faculty that consisted of two graduate teachers, one Art and one Drama, and me! It was surreal. It was incomparable to anything I was familiar with in teaching. I was not trained to teach Science or English, let alone be the faculty leader for Science! I decided that I would fake it until I made it, as teaching these subjects was temporary, with something more worthwhile and hopefully more rewarding on its way.

When I began teaching at this new school, I quickly realised that some of the teaching staff were struggling with the students. One of my

Science graduates was clearly not coping. My classroom was next to hers and I was not only observing my students, but the adventures of hers as well. There were three exit doors to her classroom and her students were running in and out of every single one of them! These little Year 7's were the kings of their own school and behaved with a fearlessness and disrespect for their new educational home, unlike anything I had ever seen in teaching before. Belligerent, defiant, empowered and completely out of control, they were physically destroying their brand-new school building. Two school cleaners, exasperated by the rapid destruction to the new classroom sliding doors and blackboard ledges that had already been torn off the walls, bailed me up to vent their distress at the end of my very first day at this school. I remember driving home like a deer in headlights thinking, *what on earth have I done?* I had gone from the frying pan and dived straight into the fire.

However, this new teaching role wasn't meant to be. I only lasted a few days in this position. By the time I began my new role, my lupus had deteriorated to the worst state it had been in since I had been diagnosed with lupus fifteen years before. I collapsed at home one morning, when I should have been getting up and ready to go to school. I couldn't lift myself out of bed. I had no strength, no energy – just pain, fatigue and fever. My mouth was covered in huge lupus-induced canker sores. I was in tears. They would not stop flowing. All of the usual lupus suspects had arrived. None of my medications could save me from this flare.

It took me eighteen months to recover. Eighteen months of unemployment and government sickness benefits. Eighteen months of combatting pain, fatigue, anger, frustration and fear. Anger was the toughest challenge to overcome, for all of the anguish of how distressing it had been for me, being bullied at my previous school, came pouring out of me. Anger over the fact that I had to leave my permanent position at this school – not the bullies. That I was not supported during those years from the administration, despite my very early attempts to seek support from them. That they knew how sick I was and yet they left me to languish and eventually deteriorate.

I felt frustration, as I had come such a long way in being true to myself and disclosing with co-workers that I had lupus, compared with my early teaching years. Frustration because I knew within a few months of beginning at that school this was not going to be the right environment for me to work in. I knew my lupus was going to deteriorate if I stayed. Frustration because I searched constantly to find another job during all of those years that I endured such a stressful work environment. I did try so hard to take care of myself. Frustration that hardly anyone I worked with really understood how serious lupus is and, worse, didn't wish to truly know, that those who I worked with, didn't care how seriously ill I was, or that their behaviour and treatment of me, was detrimental to my health.

The anger rose up from my heart, because I was now so ill from working with these women, that my lupus was made that much worse, and I was now facing the real threat of possible damage to any one of my vital organs. I felt anger and frustration because I didn't have the compassion I longed for and deserved, which cultivated the fear I now endured from the uncertainty I was experiencing, while knowing that these women, these bullies, continued teaching at the school I did love and enjoyed so much, and that they continued to thrive, while I was now on the sidelines, unsure of my teaching future and my health at rock bottom.

* * *

Thankfully, my health eventually improved with the help of all of my medications, rest, slow, incremental bouts of walking, strengthening exercises and much love from my family and friends. In time, I was able to find a teaching position that became a permanent one. But it too, has been a teaching experience fraught with more challenging, difficult and confrontational colleagues and hardships. In retrospect, despite persevering and trying to focus on the positive, worthy attributes of people like these, it eventually becomes apparent that no matter how many times you experience disappointing incidents and try to find a way forward with forgiveness, they cannot be completely overcome.

No professional or personal growth can occur, for there is no respect, no trust and no joy when you are working with selfish, aggressive and arrogant people. It becomes truly hopeless. And when you have an incurable, chronic autoimmune disease like lupus, it is unforgiveable to even waste time in trying to achieve the impossible when working in such a toxic environment. So, sadly, I have left schools when I have had these stressful experiences, even when I did not wish to, as the quality of my life needed to be the centre of my being. It is incumbent on me to spend the energy and strength I do have, working in a supportive, inclusive and caring environment.

Every time I visit my amazing rheumatologist, she reiterates the importance of no stress for me. It is so vital for Lupus Warriors to try and manage stress as best they can, particularly when it comes to the workplace. We spend so much time each day of our lives in the workplace, so we need to make sure that we are not under additional duress. We are already suffering enough. But finding the right job when you have lupus, is really hard. You need opportunity for rest, preferably each day, so that you can manage your lupus the best way you can. The regular intervals of school holidays have helped me to rest and rejuvenate, even though much of this time is spent preparing for lessons and marking assignments. But not every job provides time to have a little break like teaching does. And that's tough.

Stress causes lupus to flare. I have experienced some of the worst lupus flares as a result of stress, specifically ongoing work-related stress. I have found that reducing stress is the hardest aspect of managing my lupus. When I have worked with selfish, confrontational personalities, people that will not change their behaviour, no matter how much intervention, my heart has always suffered. When my heart is hurting, my feelings and emotions have always decided the severity of my lupus symptoms. Relationship issues with family and friends will also bring the same response. The experience of grief when someone I love passes away or when someone I love is suffering and experiencing their own health battles. Or the pain of romantic love, particularly the suffering from a broken heart, dejected and wallowing in my own loneliness. Lupus cannot always be kept under control, no matter how many pills I pop; it will always emerge as the victor. Because life is happening to me. And I cannot control my life. None of us can. For who knows what each day will bring for us?

For me, that's where the frustration comes in. The frustration of working against a tide of relentless stress that doesn't let up. Stress that I have not actively sought for myself, that I have not wished to be involved in. I have found it truly exasperating, because when I have experienced stress over a chronic, intense period of time that I cannot improve or change, I know that my lupus will suffer, no matter what I do.

No matter how hard I have tried to take care of myself, whether it be taking my medication regularly, resting during each day, trying to relax and breathe through yoga, meditation and massage, the impact of stress on my lupus has always resulted in nasty, lingering flares from which I have been slow to recover. It is frustrating, as it matters so much to me that I am living the best life I can with lupus. I am implementing every single recommendation from my rheumatologist in my daily battle to take care of myself. It matters to me because self-reflection is critical in the effective management of this incurable disease. This disease has no end date for me or for any other Lupus Warriors. For me, I need to feel at peace at the end of each day, knowing that I have done my very best to take care of myself and to keep myself in the best health possible, no matter the external forces that permeate my life. That I have made that day count. So, I get a little angry when stress and the challenges of daily life, make my lupus worse and create a dent in all of the positivity and goodwill I am trying to nurture in my disease-ridden body.

I have experienced two periods of extended sick leave in my twenty-year teaching career, where I have been extremely ill and needed to stop teaching indefinitely. Working with difficult colleagues has been the dominant cause, but in addition to that, the vocation of teaching I have pursued and revelled in vigorously has sadly become a profession where more importance is levelled at the expediency of administrative duties than the welfare and education of students. The workload has increased exponentially over the years. So much focus is now directed at the teacher, specifically blaming of the teacher for any irregularities and failings in the progression of student achievement. This is regardless of how much longer teachers are working during and after school hours. In the last few years, it has been heartbreaking to watch happy, healthy and professional teachers, crumble and burn out, effectively quitting the teaching profession altogether. When I have seen seemingly physically strong and healthy teachers struggling to cope with the demands of the job, I realise that I have done extremely well to teach at all.

However, the Department of Education's focus on so many requirements such as self-analysing the effectiveness of my teaching through rigorous, relentless, year-long staff appraisals, and its current obsession with recording and analysing data of how my students are progressing, has taken away the time and joy I used to spend researching and creating more fun, interactive activities for my students. Whether it be sitting in so many staff meetings that focus on school marketing strategies and politics in the development of numerous unclear and unnecessary leading teacher positions of responsibility; that focus on how our school curriculum excels in using information technology better than other schools, or the focus on how we as teaching staff need to continually work harder when student performance is compared to our neighbouring schools, has left me feeling disillusioned on where this vocation of mine is heading.

This type of stress is just as significant as the stress from working with colleagues that bully, let alone the ever-hormonal and increasingly anti-social behaviour of today's adolescents. Regardless of how much I love teaching, the patience, understanding and forgiveness that is needed to respond to disciplining students and reinforcing their engagement in the classroom is, on its own, exhausting, and unfortunately, being scrutinised more than ever.

I worry that I am not well enough to keep meeting these ever-changing demands in my career. Having lupus and teaching is not going to be a combination that I can sustain for much longer, if at all. Stress in the workplace will make it tougher for me to keep bouncing back from repeated lupus flares, particularly as I am getting older. And I question whether teaching is worth my perseverance, no matter how competent I am at it, no matter how much joy it brings me, no matter who I work with. Having lupus means that I am constantly playing the long game – the long game of knowing I am living life well. Hopefully, a long life. Earning an income and forging ahead in a much-loved career is integral to how this game of life is played. And in this long game, I must make sure that I am playing with people who play fair, who play with compassion, who play with kind, loving hearts. Because my long game depends on it. My life depends on it.

Chapter Twenty

Are You Really My Friend?

Whilst the relationships and friendships I have forged in my faculty area during my teaching career have often been challenging, it has been the friendships I have made with teachers outside of my faculty, that have given me the strength and comfort I have needed to endure the difficult times I've experienced as a teacher. Teachers understand each other. We speak the same language. We understand the personal and emotional demands of our roles as educators, particularly the diplomacy that is needed to overcome the often petty, vacuous politics that underpins our profession. To have met other teachers along the way who have similar values and teaching philosophies as me has been such a comfort. They have seen how much teaching means to me and the dedication I give, despite my lupus battle. They do not judge or criticise me for giving my best; they know that I love teaching and that my achievements in being well enough to teach, matter.

To have then developed few but genuine, long-lasting friendships has been an absolute gift. It's been so reassuring to know that there have been friends I could seek support from whenever I have experienced a stressful moment with either a co-worker or student/parent issue. Even better, they have taken much interest in my health and the management of my lupus. They have given me sage words of advice when I have found it difficult to look forward and overcome the frustration of working with people who are selfish and are not likely to change anytime soon. Always guiding me back to my number one priority – putting myself first and reducing stress in the management of my lupus.

If only all Lupus Warriors had supportive, understanding and non-judgemental friends who can help them to stand stronger. Despite the beautiful friendships I have made, the heartbreak from friendships that don't endure has been, at times, devastating. Unfortunately, lupus has always been at the core of their demise. I am not alone, as many Lupus Warriors and those who battle chronic illness, experience friendships that don't last. The inability of people to truly see the struggle, suffering even, which I fight through each day with lupus, often means that friendships are difficult to sustain. It is often the friends I have thought would be the most supportive that are the most disappointing. Conversely, and more positively, it is the friendships that have developed from acquaintances that have often been the sweetest surprise of all. They have helped to soften the hurt from those who have let me down.

The friendships I have lost along the way, have often been due to the inability of my friend to truly understand the chronic nature of my lupus symptoms. That is, I have an incurable disease that needs to be monitored and treated with toxic medication. Indefinitely. Some friends need to be constantly reminded of the symptoms I experience, such as joint pain, fatigue and sun-sensitivity. I have had friends who, after many years, I still needed to remind that I cannot be out in the direct rays of UV or the sun – ever! I have also had friends to whom I have had to quietly and calmly repeat, until I couldn't be bothered anymore, that I must have an afternoon nap – every single day for the foreseeable future. That this routine does not change, for I am so tired at this stage of the day, no matter how well I appear to be doing.

I have had friends who could not quite understand that even though I was working, it was medication such as steroids and methotrexate that were giving me my wings in being strong enough to work, that me being well enough to teach with lupus has been, and still is, something to be admired in recognising all of the Lupus Warriors who are too ill to work. I have had friends that have never really made me feel that they truly understand what lupus is. Friends who rarely ring me or text me to see how I am doing, even just to say, 'Hey, how are doing? Are you well? Thinking of you.' Even though I have lupus, the eventual realisation that it appears that I am hardly in their thoughts sits too heavily and uncomfortably in my heart. And I find that hard. Ultimately, I am likely to retreat and slowly drift away.

I believe that the foundation of true friendship should be unconditional care and support. I have been naïve at times to think and assume that when people learn that I have lupus, as my friend, they would reach out to me a little more frequently. Simply because I am ill and I need a little more care than most, as you would for someone battling a chronic health issue. I believe that when you are chronically ill, when you are hurt or experience disappointment, the ache in your heart becomes deeper, as you are already wounded and exposed to loss. I long for people to simply be gentle with me. I often can't believe it when friends who say they love and care for me haven't checked in to see how I am travelling more often than normal, particularly when I have been very unwell, to at least try and protect me from more disappointment when I am already so ill.

I say this because I am in tears when I watch stories about people with chronic illnesses who receive the most beautiful love and support from their family and friends. Particularly, their friends, who always rally around them when they are in need. I know how lucky I am to have the unconditional love and support from my immediate family and close friends, but when I see people who are ill, who have friends that do everything they can to help their sick friend to feel supported and less isolated, I am moved to tears. People who raise money for the illness that is affecting their friend, they give so much of their time to ensure that their sick friend never feels forgotten. It just gets to me.

Many of my friends, particularly outside of teaching, have married and had children over the years. And I have not. That alone is cause for single people like me to feel left out of the loop more and more over time. But the fact that I have been seriously ill as well has made it more difficult to swallow when my friends have started to move in different social circles and find other friends who mirror their lives. It is hurtful to be left out of group catch-ups where everyone invited is a wife and mother.

The only way forward, is to sit with the lupus experience itself – inside all of its teachings – and to find the resolve to stay true to myself in not tolerating being treated like this. Life is too short when you have lupus. Your mortality is front and centre in everything you give your heart and mind to. I have become much better in judging people when making friendships over the years. Just as importantly, I have become more comfortable walking away from friendships when I am feeling uncared for and, at times, forgotten, even when I am doing all of the reaching out, organising catch-ups and checking in with 'how are you?' The unconditional support for me is simply not there. I owe myself a good life more than ever because of my ill health. I am not going to waste my time on people who don't take care of me, like I am trying to take care of them, friends who hurt my feelings, bruise my heart or disappoint me and continue to let me down. Having lupus is doing that already. I don't need to add to my daily battle, by holding on to people who despite what they may think and feel of their contribution to our friendship, simply don't care for me in the way that I need. I would rather be alone.

* * *

Despite the friendships that don't provide the love and support we hope for as Lupus Warriors, I believe we must also be very wary of a different type of friendship that can appear without warning, often when we are sick and vulnerable and our defences are down. Beware of the 'do-gooder'. What is a do-gooder? My self-described definition of a do-gooder is someone who calls themselves your 'friend' but who is the complete opposite to whom I was describing earlier. They make it their mission to excessively seize on the opportunity to show kindness when you are ill. And they make sure that everyone knows about the goodwill they are giving you. I recommend that Lupus Warriors try to stay away from these friendships, for these people can be cunning as they try to disempower and control you when you lack the strength to be able to take care and stand up for yourself. In many ways, they exhibit narcissistic traits as it seems that all they are interested in is using your illness to better themselves in the eyes of others. I have no doubt that they are likely to puff their chests out, satisfied with their moment to shine as a caring, thoughtful soul. It is something I cannot stand. One of the few things in life that truly angers me – watching someone prey upon your pain and suffering in order to boost their own self-worth and social standing.

Unfortunately, one has to experience the workings of a do-gooder to see their true intentions. It's likely to be when you are feeling weak and extremely unwell. They may seem genuine enough by sending a card or flowers, but they also make sure that other people are included in this sentiment of kindness, for they like to be seen and revered for their thoughtfulness as the instigator and organiser of this gift.

The do-gooder may also insist on visiting you when you are home sick and bedridden. When I say insist, I mean refuse to take no for an answer. Of course, other people are aware of their impending visit for they may have told everyone at work or in your friendship circle that they intend on visiting you at home. Despite thanking them for their concern, when you express that you are not well enough for visitors at that time, that you are not well enough to socialise, they are likely to become pushy and may even bully you and offer alternative ways to visit you, insisting that they won't intrude your space.

In one case, I wasn't well enough for visitors and it took all of my strength to repeatedly tell this person that I was not well enough to get out of bed. I felt pressured, somewhat bullied, as I had to combat every alternative scenario this person was asking me to consider, saying 'But I want to come and see you,' or 'It will just be a quick visit', and so on. This person struggled to understand the meaning of the word 'no', let alone that being bedridden actually meant being bedridden. I didn't feel respected or understood and I resented being harassed in this way.

I then began to recognise something was amiss when the do-gooder, my supposed friend, didn't answer when they eventually realised that 'no, thank you' meant just that. There weren't any kind reply messages, such as, 'No worries, Rachel. Take care of yourself and I hope you are feeling better soon.' There was no reply at all. I heard nothing but silence. And it was deafening.

For I had said no, I had disempowered this person, denying them of that moment to shine brightly amidst the admiration of others for their acts of kindness. The urgency in visiting me at my worst was suddenly gone and what was leftover felt empty, disingenuous and, in some ways, cruel.

I have experienced a few similar instances like this during my time as a Lupus Warrior and I have come to be very wary of the intentions of people like this. People who are pushy and forceful. Once the do-gooder has performed their kind deed, I have found that they are not likely to even reach out to you in a few days or a week or so to see if you are feeling better. In fact, they don't reach out to you at all. And that is when you know that this person, who claimed to be your friend is, in fact, a do-gooder. For a good friend, a true friend, will always know what you need when you have lupus. They are not boasting to all and sundry of the kind deeds they are doing for you. They will rally around you in the most respectful, loving, unconditional way, during periods of both good and bad health. They will not be forceful or stroppy when you are too sick to see them. They will listen to you. They will care for you and always check in with you to see how you are. You will be in their thoughts, for they will truly love you. And, when you find these friends, these rare but true gems, you will hold them in your heart dearly, for they are Lupus Warriors too.

Chapter Twenty-One

Here Comes the Sun

'Here comes the sun … it's alright'. An iconic Beatles song often comes to mind for me when I think of the sun. Such a positive message of reassurance, that everything will be okay when the sun comes out. But sadly, for those of us who suffer sun-sensitivity with lupus, it means the complete opposite for us. It is not alright when we see the sun breaking through the sky. For me, after the initial excitement of seeing the hope of a lovely, sunny day ahead, fear quickly sets in. I start to think of what I have to do, in making sure that I am safe from the harm it will cause me, if I am standing in its glory for too long.

As I mentioned earlier in Part 2, the challenges of completing outdoor activities such as strolling through the school grounds doing yard duty can make me a very sick lady. I can walk very briskly across the school yard or down the street for a few minutes or so, but standing, front and centre for five minutes or longer in the direct rays of the sun, can cause a thumping headache, butterfly rash across my face, a fever and fatigue. It's a scary feeling when I experience this. I can feel the heat of the sun penetrating on my head and face, and then the pulsing starts, with pain and sleepiness not far behind. So quick and intense that I just long to shut my eyes and fall asleep. And I realise, I just have to move. Immediately. To find retreat under cover or indoors. To be safe.

If I haven't been quick enough, or if the UV rays are at their peak, the sun can trigger a full-on lupus flare. One of the lupus flares I have experienced out of the blue, was when I made the risky decision one morning to hang some washing on the line on a sunny day. I reassured myself that it would only take a couple of minutes and that I should be okay. Well, those few minutes caused a lot of damage. I was off school for three weeks with one of the worst lupus flares I had experienced in a long time. All of my medicines were increased, particularly the steroids, to reduce the inflammation in my body, which would in turn reduce my pain and fatigue. It was a very difficult flare to bounce back from, particularly when I was missing so many classes with my senior students. Catching up and getting my students back on track was relentless and didn't give me much room for convalescing. It took me months to get my lupus back under control.

Cloudy days can cause just as much damage, particularly if the UV ray coverage is strong. So, outdoor activities, sunny or cloudy, must be addressed with the same preventative measures: UV50+ sunscreen on my face, neck and exposed arms and legs; protective clothing; floppy hat and sunglasses.

According to the Lupus Foundation of America, 40% to 70% of lupus patients will find that their lupus is made worse by exposure to UV rays from sunlight and artificial light.[17] That is a large number of people affected. Artificial light can also cause lupus flares. Aside from the elements of UV ray damage from the sun, Lupus Warriors become photosensitive. This means that items such as UV fluorescent lights, under prolonged exposure, are another trigger for a flare. When I sit under a reading lamp, within ten minutes my face starts to turn red and flushed; my butterfly rash spreading its harmful wings.

So why are people with lupus so sensitive to the sun, to UV rays and UV fluorescent lights? According to the Lupus Foundation of America, exposure to UV light causes damage to everyone's cellular DNA. This is called UV radiation and occurs regardless of whether it's coming from the sun or a lamp. In people with lupus, the cells are much more sensitive to the damage caused by UV radiation. Normally, the immune system clears damaged cells, but in people with lupus, these cells are cleared more slowly. The dead cells stick around in the body, which can then trigger an immune system attack, such as a lupus flare.

Adding to the risk of lupus flares from the sun's rays and UV fluorescent light, are the major medications that many Lupus Warriors take on a daily, indefinite basis. Medications such as anti-inflammatory drugs, the anti-malarial hydroxychloroquine, the immunosuppressant methotrexate and even some antibiotics. Being photosensitive is already compounded with so many risks from the physical environment but to also be at risk because of our medicines as well is a real blow.

It's fair to say that at times, I've felt extremely frustrated by the limitations I have being photosensitive. Aside from the ongoing challenges of navigating a safe place for me to be in the workplace, away from the harmful UV rays of the sun outdoors, teaching in classrooms that have numerous UV fluorescent lights glaring down on me each day has always been an ongoing issue. There are so many of these artificial lights in the classroom. So often, I leave the classroom completely red-faced, feverish, head-aching and tired. If I am already at risk of flaring, I stand no chance if I am in these classrooms for too long.

Even after thirty years, my acceptance of being photosensitive is still tested during social occasions that should bring joy and happiness. Instead, I often find myself fighting back tears of sorrow. Whether it be barbeques, weddings or outdoor birthday gatherings, I am trapped within the confines of hiding from the sun. I can't stand and talk and laugh where most of my friends are gathered. I have to find the safe spot that will shield me from harm. At these events, you will find me standing awkwardly under pergolas, deckings or super shady trees, trying desperately to fit in with my wide-brimmed floppy hat and sunnies. Looking happy and relaxed is the aim, but inside, I am stressed, frustrated and fearful. I am likely to last only minutes like this, with the power of those rays so strong, they will find a way to creep in and reach me, even under cover.

So ultimately, I will end up indoors, seated uncomfortably in a lounge or kitchen area, chatting to an elderly uncle or neighbour of the party thrower who I haven't met before, isolated from the happy moments and memories being created amongst my friends, outside in the beautiful sunshine. Often, when my mates are having a good time, many of them forget about my sun-sensitivity (which I know sounds so strange to them, simply because they don't remember that it is a huge issue for me) and are not always willing to make sacrifices in being with me to help me feel more comfortable. Only true friends will do this for me. Forgive me for whining, but it can feel so cruel to watch others be so joyous and carefree in the somewhat simple act of just basking in the sunshine and with each other. How I long to be them. Depending on how I am feeling, I will either persevere and stay or I will leave early, fighting back tears as I struggle to relax and truly enjoy myself.

Over the years, I simply feel tired at the thought of those feelings and frustrations returning when I am invited to special occasions that are in the outdoors. I am likely to decline. It's just easier. Less stressful, less heartbreaking for me.

It's not just big social events like these that cause such angst. Regular activities in daily life need to be modified to enable me to be out in the world, protected from the sun. Sitting close to windows in cafés is a no-no, as the UV penetrates the glass. I am at risk even inside, even on a cloudy day. So, I always try and sit deep inside the café, up the back and rarely outdoors. It can be an issue when I am out and about with friends. My quiet, no-fuss sensibilities are challenged as I must be assertive and find my voice in asking to be seated in an area where I can be protected. Day trips to sporting events are out. I miss going to the footy during the day, but I can go at night, which, in the end, is all that matters.

Going on holiday can be a challenge. There is no frolicking on the sand or in the water during the day for me. That's hard for people I am on holiday with, who long to do that. But I can wait until the sun goes down and make my way into the water then. It may be cooler, darker and for a shorter period of time, but at least I am at the beach – in the moment.

One of the biggest aspects of being photosensitive that has required the most adaptation is my love of gardening. I can't tell you how depressed and frustrated I get when a beautiful sunny day, temperature at low to mid-twenties arrives and I hear the sound of lawn mowers and whipper snippers buzzing. Knowing that other people are outside in their gardens, enjoying the sun, the fresh air and the earth between their fingers … that's heaven for me. Knowing I can't join them, leaves me feeling bereft.

Fortunately, there are other ways I can garden. It just means a smaller amount of time for me and its likely to be at the end of the day, after 5.30 pm, when the sun is going down. This can be challenging too, as I have an afternoon nap each day, which can eat into the time I could be spending outside in the garden! The frustration of fighting off pesky mosquitoes and other flying bugs that thrive at this time of night can be worrying. I mustn't get bitten, as I am at risk of infection due to being completely immunosuppressed. Having lupus is indeed a risky business!

So, you will find me during these garden-friendly evenings, lathered up in Aero guard, enjoying the earth between my fingers, but in the dark. It's not the same as a gorgeous sunny day but it's the closest I can get in being able to enjoy my garden. Because it offers such a small window of time, I revel in being there, cherishing what I am able to do, despite the limitations lupus has delivered. Finding perspective in these moments is really important for many Lupus Warriors who are also photosensitive, like me. We need to reduce stress to help keep our lupus under control. If I am feeling stressed and focusing on what I can't do, I am not helping myself at all. Finding hope in all that I can do, has given me the insight I need when I am feeling the pain and frustration of having lupus. Having a good sook is so important too! I try to remind myself that it is okay to miss my pre-lupus life.

I try not to sit in these tears for too long, for I must keep making every day count. I remember the humorous moments that being photosensitive has brought me. There was one occasion when I was getting my hair washed at the hair salon by a hair dressing apprentice. Out of the blue, she said, 'I really love the blush you are wearing. What is it called?' I wanted to burst out laughing. I have never worn blush in my life! The blush this poor girl was referring to was the red butterfly rash that was spread gently across my cheeks. Not wanting to embarrass her, I replied, 'It's an organic brand.' She seemed happy with that answer! Less humorous was the time I was berated by a work colleague for getting sunburnt over the weekend. Again, my face was covered in a particularly deep, red butterfly rash. It really did look like I was sunburnt. She absolutely ripped into me about how foolish I had been in not covering up when in the sun. When I finally had a chance to get a word in, I quietly explained to her what it was, much to her dismay. She was quite an opinionated, judgemental lady, so it was a good opportunity for her to learn that not everything appears to be what it seems.

When the sun is shining down, I take pleasure in knowing the joy that it does bring to us all; I need to remember that although it feels like my enemy at times, it is shining a light on me in a different way. A special way.

LUPUS = Lift Up, Persevere, Use Strength

For it is showing me that the small doses of sunlight I do have exposure to are to be savoured. Treasured. And that, for me, is a life hopefully being lived well.

Chapter Twenty-Two

But Do You Know? Do You Really Know?

Over the years, I've come to liken the feeling of battling lupus, to the principles of the board game Snakes and Ladders, which I referred to earlier. When the dice rolls, you take the number of steps forward that the dice dictates. Literally, one step at a time. When you are feeling well and your lupus is under control, you may even land on a ladder and climb up the board that little bit further. When that is happening, you feel truly happy, as you are able to maintain a sense of balance and stability. It just feels good. But then the game can change, on its head without warning and that dice can roll toward that snake. When you hit that snake, it boldly raises its head and hisses at you. Taunting you. Because, you know what is coming. For you have suffered another setback, another lupus flare. And so, you begin to slide. You slide all the way down the back of that slippery snake, sometimes to the bottom of the board. That soaring happiness dissipates, as you realise that you have to begin the game all over again and fight your way back up to the top of the board. This is how the game of lupus is played. Over and over and over again. At some point, you will always fall back down. Why? Because lupus always wins.

So, the never-ending tweaking of medication takes place, whether it be increased steroids or methotrexate, which will then require months and months of tapering back to the dose at which you were originally controlling your lupus, before that flare took you down. It can be draining. Bloody frustrating. Particularly when I have felt as though I was managing my lupus and overall health, with all of my ducks in a row and then, *boom!* A flare can happen for any reason at all. Stress is most likely to be the usual culprit, but infections, exposure to UV rays or changes in the weather can also be to blame. It also flares up, simply because it can.

Often when I'm flaring, I feel overwhelmed with all of the disruption that the lupus flare is bringing. I keep everything in perspective but it can be hard. As a senior schoolteacher, I have been agitated at the thought of all of the work that needs to be done to keep my students on track whilst I've been absent, not to mention the huge work load that awaits me when I get back to school. On the plus side, because I know I am susceptible to unexpected flares, I have most lessons organised and ready to go. However, the communication, particularly by email, to my replacement teacher and students whilst I am flaring, can be exhausting. It becomes difficult to switch off at the best of times as a teacher, but when you are ill and your students are depending on you, the weight of these responsibilities feels relentless.

When I have these worries swirling in my head, I know I am not helping myself to heal my flare. I realise that the only way to fight back, is to simply let go. Let go of everything. Place myself in a protective bubble and completely shut down. To focus on myself. Hope that the drugs kick in quickly and move with the pain and discomfort the best way I can. I feel accepting that I am battling something far greater than myself, is critical in how well I will manage this disease. As a Lupus Warrior, I must respect what this disease is and what it can do. If I wage a war against myself and push through without enough rest and respite, I will be causing more inflammation, more damage to my body. And that is no good for me in the short or long term, for I am managing a disease that is unlikely to be leaving me anytime soon.

I need to be gentle with myself. To be kind to myself. If that means having a teary and a good sook, so be it. If that means I am in bed for days or even weeks, I have no choice but to give in. If it means I am back on the high doses of steroids and methotrexate, with all of the nasty side effects that come with these drugs, then that's just the way it is. I have to just roll with it as best I can. I need to let go so that I can get back on that game board again and keep rolling the dice.

* * *

It's the loss of potential earnings that can be quite devastating. It can be very difficult to save for a house deposit or special holiday when so much of my income goes towards the expense of medications, doctor's appointments and pathology tests. It's not just the cost of all of the heavy medications that hits my back pocket, it's all of the creams, eye drops, vitamins and mineral supplements that I need to treat all of the ongoing deficiencies, such as iron and calcium, and conditions such as Sjogren's syndrome, which I have developed, because I have lupus. I feel as though I am always dragging myself off to the chemist. When I am struggling financially, I am ashamed to say that I have at times, compromised my health by not purchasing items that can ease my discomfort. I tell myself that I can get by for a few days longer without those eye drops. I can cope with the dryness, the grittiness just a little longer. I have no doubt that many fellow Lupus Warriors would know what I am talking about here.

It can get that tough, particularly when I'm living on my own. I make these decisions, these sacrifices, to simply cope and to make sure I have enough money to pay the bills. Despite feeling distraught during these times, the blessings are there to be realised. I am so fortunate to have access to all of these medications. It doesn't bare thinking about, not having them. I know that I would not be able to live the quality of life I have without them.

So much loss can be experienced by those with lupus and other chronic autoimmune diseases in regard to their career earnings and accumulating a decent amount of their superannuation. My health has deteriorated in recent years. In 2013, I developed a condition called fibromyalgia (I will discuss this in the next chapter). It has resulted in a slow decline in the amount of days I am able to work. When I started teaching, I managed to work full-time. After ten years of teaching full-time, I slowly dropped to working for four and half days a week, then four, and then eventually the equivalent of three days a week, spread out over the working week.

Fortunately for me, I had reached the top of the teaching pay scale, so the income I was earning for three days a week was just enough for me to live on. If I was teaching three days a week in my graduate teaching years, I would have been in trouble. It has been quite a strain to manage financially working these reduced hours. I have also had periods when I have had to stop teaching for about a month or two prior to the end of the school year to simply rest and keep my lupus under control. I had to take six months off school, when I was diagnosed with fibromyalgia in 2013.

Battling an autoimmune disease like lupus, I have had barely any sick leave up my sleeve. Working part-time, I have hardly received any sick leave at all, due to the small-time fraction I have been working. I use up all of my sick days every year, and then some. I've lost hundreds and hundreds of dollars over the years, due to taking sick leave without pay when I have had no sick leave days left to use. It's gut-wrenching, particularly when I have been really ill and my pay for the next few fortnights plummets to next to nothing.

Worst of all, after twenty years of teaching, I've never been able to take long service leave to go on a special holiday or simply take a break. I've only ever taken long service leave so that I can go on sick leave because I have run out of days to be paid. This has been the only solution, so that I could survive financially. I've been hesitant to access my superannuation to keep me going, but it's there if I desperately need it. The long-service leave I do have left must sit there untouched, waiting to be used to keep me afloat when I am ill again. I am not alone with these battles and worries, but at least I have been able to work. At least I have had access to a financial solution, when I am feeling so ill. My heart breaks for all of the Lupus Warriors who are too ill to work at all or ever. They rely on government welfare and the charity of loved ones to survive.

* * *

Having lupus or any incurable disease, comes with such physical loss. Loss in so many different shapes and forms. For me, my mind can let me down. I can get so confused, truly scrambled when attempting the most menial and simplest of tasks. Having lupus can cause a phenomenon called 'lupus fog'. Being on all of these heavy medications, particularly methotrexate, intensifies these symptoms. It's an apt name to describe this sensation, as I do feel so foggy and unclear. I've had so many terrifying moments where I cannot, for the life of me, remember where I have parked my car when I am out at shopping centres or at the market. I genuinely think at the time, that it has been stolen. Re-tracing my steps is challenging when I am like this. Fear, panic and distress intertwine and stop me from focusing on trying to remember any surrounding landmarks or objects that may trigger my memory. The relief and elation of finally figuring out where my car is, is expressed with both joy and tears. I can't help but feel a little sorry for myself. I've often found that when I am like this, I am either really fatigued or a lupus flare is coming.

My lupus fog experiences have deteriorated in recent years. I'm constantly walking into rooms, not knowing why I am there. If I do remember something that needs to be done, I find that I cannot hold that thought. I have to write it down immediately or that thought will be gone. Struggling to spell simple, everyday words can sneak into my daily practice. Sometimes, I have forgotten the names of people at school, particularly my students. This can be both embarrassing and scary. My students have constantly corrected me when I have made mistakes on the board. I have often written the same word twice or forgotten to write key words or full sentences. I use humour to cope during these moments, but inside, I'm really embarrassed.

I find that some administrative tasks at work become difficult to complete. I can believe that I have met a school deadline, but then learn that I haven't. Or I can get deadlines mixed up in my head, completing them at the wrong times. On one occasion, I didn't show up for an exam supervision I was scheduled to take. I misunderstood the instructions and went to supervise a different exam! (On reflection, what was truly worrying, is that it took the staff supervising this exam well over forty minutes to realise that I shouldn't have even been there!)

For a conscientious, organised person like me, it can be very upsetting when I make mistakes like these at work. I can become inconsolable with myself, particularly at the thought of making a bigger mistake that could negatively impact on someone else, such as the exam mishap. I don't want to let anyone down. It's difficult to explain to people at work that I am experiencing this because, to them, I look and sound fine. My distress, my lupus, is invisible to them.

The best practice I can use in trying to navigate life in a lupus fog is to write everything down. Sticky notes are everywhere on my desk at work and at home. When it becomes overwhelming looking at all of these notes laying everywhere, I take stock and try to actually do the things I have written down and reminded myself to do. It's hard because these tasks are likely to be building up and left undone because I'm not feeling well. If I am parking my car in a different place from normal, I write down the level or landmarks that will help me remember (but, I do have to remind myself to do this, which is the problem!) In general, I just have to move through these moments without judgement. I must keep reminding myself that it's not my fault, that I am not purposefully trying to make mistakes or upset anyone. Creating more stress and frustration for myself will not help me to move forward.

* * *

I have moments, particularly when I am feeling a little flat and am struggling more than usual, when I find myself in grief for the physical form that I used to be. The disease itself, and the use of drugs during these last thirty years, decides what physical shape my body will take, regardless of how well I eat or how much I exercise. Taking steroids has had the most significant impact, particularly during my delicate, teenage years. They have changed who I am and what I look like. Now, at the age of forty-four, I still have scars from those tumultuous years of increased, intense steroid doses. These scars are mainly on my legs; permanent reminders of that time and the intensity of my young growing body being stretched to capacity. I also have so much fluid retention in my back, stomach and behind my knees that just won't shift. I try not to be too vain, but I can't help it sometimes, as I'm a little curious as to what my body would look like if I didn't have lupus or if I didn't have to take all of these drugs.

Thankfully, perspective and gratitude eventually put me back into my place, as I concede that I am simply lucky to be managing as well as I have, for as long as I have. That I can honestly say I have done my best to look after myself, particularly in regard to diet and exercise. And that just has to be enough.

More seriously, after nearly twenty years of taking steroids, I had to stop taking them. I had developed a condition in my bones called osteopenia. Osteopenia is one step away from full-blown osteoporosis, which is a disease in the bones that leaves the bones porous, fragile and susceptible to breakage.

Taking steroids for that long, on reflection, is a good innings. I've read so many stories where some people with lupus have had to stop taking steroids within a year of taking them because they have developed full-blown osteoporosis. A calcium-enriched diet and good genes are likely to have helped me to go the distance. But oh, how I miss them at times. Whilst I don't miss the way they change my temperament or the additional weight gain, I miss the burst of energy and strength they provide. It's such a gift, particularly during a flare. Trying to manage without them has been a challenge, but I've adapted well, with methotrexate, Plaquenil, a hormone called DHEA and an NSAID called Mobic, now being my current drug regime.

The continual fluctuation of weight gain with the varying doses of steroids and methotrexate I have been on can be frustrating, let alone expensive. I became hopeful that I would lose all of the steroid weight I had gained over the years, when I came off them. How wrong I was! For me, methotrexate causes weight gain in equal measure. My wardrobe at home has different sizes for pants, shirts and dresses, on each of the various doses of methotrexate I have had to take. I become upset, particularly if a favourite piece of clothing doesn't fit anymore. I value my possessions – what I own and what I am able to afford. To spend money on clothing I can't wear is upsetting. No doubt for all Lupus Warriors like me.

Being a Lupus Warrior means that we are in constant fear and angst of what could be next. The threat of developing other autoimmune diseases, even cancer, is very real. As I mentioned before, when you have one autoimmune disease, there is likely to be another one that will develop as well. Lupus Warriors are at risk of developing additional autoimmune diseases such as thyroid disease, coeliac disease and rheumatoid arthritis. I'm always checking for lumps or any changes in my lupus symptoms. It's imperative that I remain vigilant and recognise any signs of change in how I am feeling and how I look. But it's so exhausting. There are so many moments, where I just want to take a break from having lupus and all of these additional worries. A time-out. Particularly after thirty years, I feel I am at least due for some annual leave. Don't you think? *(wink, wink!)*

* * *

The frustration of not being able to be of more help to people in need is a huge loss that I also struggle with. I wish I was able to participate in charity walks, donate blood and volunteer in children's hospitals, as these are things I would really love to do. To be of help to people who need it, without hesitation. To make more of a difference in this world. Then I remember, I'm in need of a little charity myself and that I'm completely immunosuppressed, which means that I am at a higher risk of infection and must be extremely careful of the environments I expose myself to. That I must seek help, accept help and focus on taking good care of myself, so that I can be of help to others, even if it's in the smallest of ways. That in itself, is making a difference. But it can still get to me, watching people who are well enough to give to others in need and the sense of purpose and joy that it brings to be able to give.

Becoming pregnant and giving birth is a challenge for female Lupus Warriors, and for many, not a possibility. Being immunosuppressed, particularly taking methotrexate, means that you cannot become pregnant whilst taking this medication. The methotrexate is too toxic. The only way a Lupus Warrior can become pregnant, if she is able, is to stop taking methotrexate or any other similar immunosuppressant medication altogether. To do this is extremely challenging, as the female Lupus Warrior is at risk of flaring without these medications, which are controlling the disease. She has to undertake the gruelling task of slowly tapering off this medication, which will make her feel pretty crappy, and somehow persevere with the hope that she can successfully conceive a child.

As I am currently completely – and indefinitely – immunosuppressed, as well as single, I fear my chances of becoming a mum, are extremely slim – particularly given my age. And for that I am so, so sad. Reaching this age has truly snuck up on me, as it does for everyone, no doubt. For whatever reason, the right man hasn't come along for me yet, or within the biological period appropriate for having a baby. I have not had the money to pop down to the sperm bank to conceive a child that way either! Now in my early forties, I am having a hard time coming to terms with where I am in my life. I've always known that having children would be difficult for me, whether it be conceiving or simply having the energy and strength needed to be a good mum. Watching my friends become mothers over the years has been lovely to watch, but also a painful reminder of what might not be for me. Particularly when mothers whinge about their child and how hard motherhood is, it's excruciating for me to listen to such comments.

The grief of watching everyone have what I perceive to be a normal life fluctuates for me. How do I rise above their happiness and normality without feeling envious or jealous of the effortlessness of their lives? Most people use language that is very definitive. Words like, 'I am going to …' and 'we are …' They have no doubts, only certainty that what they want and intend to do will be and will happen. How do I, as a Lupus Warrior, immerse myself in a world that talks like this, thinks like this, when I cannot? Everything I do hinges on how well I am, how controlled my lupus is, when each new day arrives. I am fraught with the hope that I am even well enough to be able to do what I have planned. I won't know until that new day comes.

So, I sit and watch. And listen. To my colleagues at work. My friends. To people in the cafés. And I can't help but wonder. I ask myself, do they know? Do they really know how amazing their life is? The simplicity of it. They get up for work so effortlessly each day. They are physically strong enough to work full-time every day. Do they know how lucky they are to have found their soulmate, their wife, husband or partner? To be blessed with children and a mortgage? Do they know how amazing it is that they can aim high in their career, have the ability and good health to apply for promotions and attain greater success and financial security when they achieve these aspirations? They can afford holidays regularly and travel to amazing places. Do they know how wonderful it is that they can decide on a whim what they would like to do on weeknights and weekends? That they don't have to worry about overdoing it or making sacrifices so that they can be strong enough to make it to work each day?

I know I'm generalising here and I know that what I see is not always what it seems, but when the demands of battling lupus are overwhelming me, my spirit and ability to persevere is shaken and my feelings of resentment can rise up quite strongly. And then I feel foolish for comparing my life with the lives of others, making me feel quite ashamed that I am not learning the lessons lupus is teaching me.

Maybe they do know how fortunate they are. But maybe they don't. Because their life is their normal, just like life with lupus is my normal. But at times, I can't help myself. Being immersed in the politics of daily working life can be exasperating. Listening to my colleagues whinging about the smallest, pettiest of problems or for criticising and pulling apart the virtue of another co-worker, I just want to scream at them for wasting their day, for wasting their good health, their good fortune on how great their life really is. It feels as though they don't care to find the gratitude in all that they can do and all that they have.

For me, life with lupus is a long-term grieving process. An intense grief for all of the things I cannot do or be. A persistent grief that I must co-exist with – the person that God, the universe, has destined for me to be. Watching myself suffer and struggle, at times, leaves me reeling with a yearning for the person I thought I would be. It can be difficult knowing that while you have lupus, fulfilling your true potential, may not come to be.

There are many moments when my acceptance of who I am is tested. When I have stopped having a pity party for myself, thankfully, I am now wise enough to bring myself back into line. I do know how blessed I have been to be able to teach. Period. Every moment I have had in the classroom, be it good or bad, the gift of lupus has brought me back to the realisation of how great my life actually has been. I am proud to be even able to say that I have been a teacher. I think back to all of the nay-sayers, the negative comments and people who had no faith in me or my dream to be a successful teacher. And I have to smile. Deep down, I do feel content that I have stayed true to myself, for the battle of fighting to stay strong, reducing stress and controlling disease has become greater and more important than imagining what I can truly achieve in the workplace.

Once I have stifled my sobbing and dried my tears, during those lonely moments of lamenting what might not be and what is, perspective does eventually come to land gently in my heart and thus grounds me. It's these times of reflection that provide much growth. It's a reminder that I am human – that my feelings, emotions, my heart, will always be stretched and re-shaped throughout my life. I am being taught the most valuable of lessons – to just live. To make every single day count. An acceptance that this is my life and doing my best every single day, will help me to keep finding a way forward. Despite my wistfulness, I am finding more peace with what I am able to do. And I am thankfully reminded that I am lucky to be here. Lucky to be alive. This should always be my guiding light.

But I will always miss who I thought I was going to be. Rachel Lea who doesn't have lupus. I really do miss knowing her.

Chapter Twenty-Three

Making Lemonade out of Lemons

In addition to my Snakes and Ladders analogy, I often like to imagine that controlling my lupus symptoms, is like trying to keep a wolf trapped inside a box. I say wolf because the word 'lupus' is Latin for wolf. I imagine that I am trying to do all I can through stress management, from taking my medication regularly and wellness practices, to keep this wolf trapped inside of this box, lid shut tight. When I am feeling well, it means that the wolf is neatly tucked inside the box. The lid is shut. Completely. But, when I am feeling unwell, my lupus symptoms begin to reappear with intensity. Its beastly head has found a way out and is peering outside of the box. Its claws are next, ready to strike me down. Again.

Over the last thirty years of having lupus, I feel like I have managed really well in keeping my wolf in its box. With all of the highs and lows that life has brought me, I've always tried to be steadfast in doing everything I can possibly do to keep my lupus under control. The low times are the toughest times to keep the condition in its place. As I've said previously, there is no stopping a flare when I am deeply upset or heartbroken. I've learnt to go with the flow, trying not to judge myself by being kind to myself and to work through those stressful, heart-wrenching times the best way I can.

Over the years, when those stresses don't improve, I have become better at recognising when to pull back from people causing me that stress or to leave jobs that show no signs of improving. I've become more proactive about putting my health first. As I have aged, I've become more conscious of the important responsibility I have, to make sure I am doing everything I possibly can, to be as well as I can. It means so much to me to be able to say that I am doing that every day.

The most confronting aspect of having lupus over the last thirty years, has been watching my slow decline. From working full-time in my twenties to now, forty-four years old and not working at all, is both sad and confronting. My lupus symptoms have remained relatively unchanged, but some new variations of symptoms have appeared. I have a constant butterfly rash on my face, more chronic than ever before, with strange blood sores also appearing inside and outside of my nose and face. The blood sores on my nose will not heal. I have a chronic rash on my neck and upper chest.

As shared earlier in the book, despite having perfect urine, clear of blood or protein for over twenty years, in the last ten years, traces of protein and blood have regularly appeared. Visits to kidney specialists on occasion to monitor this problem brings greater worry of how my kidneys are functioning. I seem to have a rare condition where my kidney leaks small traces of protein from time to time. Thankfully, all current signs indicate that my kidneys are healthy, but it is another reminder that lupus symptoms can change. My body can continue to become inflamed and damaged by lupus as time goes on, no matter how well I take care of myself. Therefore, I must continue to be as vigilant as ever in monitoring my health.

The Raynaud's symptoms I experience in my hands are similar to when I first experienced them at the age of fourteen. Now, together with my hands, my feet are just as cold and extremely hot. It's a strange sensation. They can be ice cold, but when they reach normal temperature to touch, they feel to me as though they are on fire. It's very difficult to get them feeling just right. The secondary Sjogren's symptoms, such as dry eyes, have intensified over the years. I rarely experience a day without sore, dry eyes, not to mention dryness in other areas. It can be draining, particularly when you are reading and completing daily tasks. Just another thing that adds to feeling unwell.

The biggest challenge since being diagnosed with lupus began in 2011. Out of the blue, I developed chronic insomnia. It was torturous. I spent night after night completely wide awake, with not a wink of sleep. At the time, I didn't feel as though I was experiencing any additional worries that would be keeping me awake. It was so strange to be both wide awake and completely exhausted at the same time. I was absolutely distraught. Teaching was impossible in this state. Sleeping tablets from my GP were not working. One night was so bad, I drove myself to the emergency ward of my local hospital to seek help. By the time I got to see a doctor, I was a mess. I said to her, 'There is something terribly wrong with me. I suffer from lupus and I cannot sleep. This is not normal.' She didn't know what to say. She wrote a prescription for another sleeping tablet, which was not effective either, and sent me on my way.

Concerned with my lack of improvement, my GP put me on stronger medication to make me sleepy. It helped me rest but I was still awake frequently throughout the night. I felt stressed and frustrated. I just knew there was something physically, not mentally, wrong with me. How on earth could I be sleepless and suffer from lupus? Lupus always wins. The fatigue it produces is normally too powerful for any mental health issues to derail what it does. I just couldn't figure out what was happening to me.

Over time, my sleep did improve. However, the quality of my sleep wasn't great and I continued to feel exhausted. It didn't take long for my lupus to start to flare, as I feared it would. I would recover from a flare, then another flare would appear soon after. School became incredibly difficult to manage and my working hours were decreased to four days a week. I battled on like this for another eighteen months.

At the end of 2012, I needed to take early leave from teaching. I finished up in early November. I was just so exhausted. During this time, I tried to rest and reduce stress, with the plan to return to teaching in the new year. During January 2013, I began to experience the most intense but transient pain in my upper back and shoulders. I say transient, because it would literally come and go. It felt strange to me, because whenever I experience pain in my upper back and shoulders during a lupus flare, that pain does not ease up and I always feel so fatigued that I can actually sleep during this pain. Then, the increased steroid and methotrexate doses begin to reduce the inflammation of the flare. Once those meds kick in, the pain subsides and I slowly, slowly start to feel more energetic, stronger and pain-free. But worryingly, this pain was different.

It was weeks before the 2013 school year was due to begin and I was not well at all. The pain in my upper shoulders and back kept recurring and intensifying. I was in bed, trying so hard to rest and not worry, but it was pointless. I knew there was no way I could return to school feeling like this. Concerned by these symptoms, my rheumatologist put me back on steroids to see if this would help ease the pain. Even though I had not taken steroids each day since 2006 due to the development of osteopenia in my bones, I have on occasion had very short courses of steroids to help treat difficult lupus flares.

Each week, the commencement date for Term 1 got closer and closer and I was still not improving. In fact, I was getting worse. The steroids were not easing my pain, despite increasing their dose. Extremely worried by my lack of improvement, my rheumatologist called me in to see her. She performed a physical examination that assessed my response to touch. I did not perform well on this test, as she confirmed her suspicion that the pain I had been suffering from was due to a condition called fibromyalgia.

Fibromyalgia is a disorder that affects the muscles and soft tissues of the body. It is often characterised by widespread and chronic muscle pain and stiffness, extreme fatigue, problems with sleep such as insomnia and painful and tender spots on the body.[18] Currently, doctors are not sure what causes fibromyalgia, but some think that it's a problem with how the brain and spinal cord process pain signals from the nerves. Other symptoms include difficulty concentrating and remembering, called 'fibro fog'; feeling nervous, worried or depressed; irritable bowel syndrome; headaches; dry mouth, nose and eyes; and frequent urination.[19]

You are at greater risk of developing fibromyalgia if you are a woman, suffer from another painful disease such as lupus or rheumatoid arthritis or if you have a mood disorder such as depression or anxiety. There is no cure for fibromyalgia but a combination of medication, exercise and management of stress may ease symptoms to the point where a normal, active life can be lived.[20]

Finally, everything began to make sense. The chronic insomnia I had experienced, increased fatigue and pain … I had been suffering from fibromyalgia, undiagnosed, for over two years. Possibly, even longer. My own suspicion that something physical was wrong with me was right.

I guess that is the problem with having fibromyalgia. Its symptoms of fatigue, muscle and joint pain mirror so many other conditions, and without blood tests to accurately confirm its diagnosis, it takes a long time to detect.

My rheumatologist informed me that I would need a few months to get both my lupus and fibromyalgia under control. I would be taking another new medicine to help treat my fibromyalgia symptoms and I needed time to adjust. My lupus had also been flaring during this time off school so I also needed to rest and recover from that. It became clear that my lupus had been quietly fighting the fibromyalgia, this new condition, for a few years. They had been at loggerheads with each other. Now, they had to learn to co-exist with one another. I had to now learn how to live with another illness. Life suddenly became even harder than ever.

I was absent from school during the first term in 2013. I did my best to focus on myself, to rest and be patient in my recovery, but it was a challenge at times. I had two Year 12 Health and Human Development (HHD) classes and they didn't have their regular teacher – me. Thankfully, a good friend of mine was available to take my place. She was able to guide my students into the new school year.

When I was feeling better, I returned to school in Term 2. However, I was to take it slowly. I was only able to teach two of my Year 12 HHD classes for the duration of 2013. That's all. My principal was extremely supportive, enabling me to come to school to teach my classes, then go home to sleep and work at my own pace. My income was extremely low but, amazingly, I managed. It was a huge learning curve for me, because whenever I was experiencing muscle pain, I always thought it was lupus. Now, with fibromyalgia in the mix, so often I just wasn't sure. I had to become used to muscular pain that was persistent yet transient and figure how far to keep going, to learn the difference between the two diseases. Even today, I'm still adjusting.

It was a huge undertaking when I returned to school. I had missed the first term, a crucial period when, as a teacher, much time is invested in establishing student-teacher rapport. I had missed that and had to work quickly to get to know all of my students. It was a difficult time, as some of my colleagues had advised me not to work too hard for my students upon my return to teaching. Their negativity was not surprising, but it still wasn't welcome or easy to hear.

In the end, my students' achievements proved to be the light at the end of the tunnel for me. They achieved some of the best results in my teaching career. One student achieved 50 out of a possible 50 and many achieved results greater than 40. Their achievements were simply outstanding. I was so humbled and extremely emotional about their success. I still am to this day.

During this challenging time, I'd never been happier knowing that my true self remained strong, despite the attempts of others to break my spirit. Unfortunately, I had experienced this in the workplace too many times before and I simply shut out their negativity, stayed positive and looked forward to seeing how high my students could soar. They were the lemonade I had helped to create out of the lemons I had been dealt with, in this change to my health. At the time, they gave me hope that I would be able and, hopefully, well enough to keep teaching.

Between 2014 and the first term of 2017, I increased my working hours to the equivalent of working three days a week. My working hours were spread out over five days and I could start later or finish earlier on some days. This was critical in being able to adapt to my new life with fibromyalgia. My subject load slightly increased as each year went on. Worryingly, I reached a point at the beginning of 2017, where I was beginning to seriously struggle with my health again. My lupus flared twice within a few weeks of each other. I knew I had landed on that long, poisonous snake and I could feel myself plummeting to the bottom of that Snakes and Ladders board.

That is where I found myself – curled up, sick and frightened. The decision of not returning to school for the remainder of 2017 was made for me. I was not strong enough to keep bouncing back. My blood tests were not great, with too much lupus activity present. I was experiencing much stress in my school environment and it was finally impacting on my health, despite my best efforts to stay positive and persevere. I was under chronic stress, which showed no signs of improving. Controlling my lupus, in addition to managing my fibromyalgia symptoms, was not going to be achievable if I didn't stop, let go and heal.

As I write this book, this is where I still am. I have not been well enough to return to the demands of teaching for the last three years or simply to even work. For the second time in my life, I am relying on government benefits and the amazing charity of my family to help me survive financially. I'm terrified of my unknown future. I have loved being a teacher. What's more, aside from the joy of watching my students achieve their true potential, I have been quietly proud to see myself grow and improve during the last twenty years I've been teaching. I have not taken any opportunities I have been given for granted. Thankfully, I have always stopped to recognise how lucky I have been to be working as a teacher – such a special gift, for knowing this has given me much comfort during this challenging time, knowing that I haven't wasted my life or the good health I have been given, in being able to reach forward in my teaching career each day. But my secondary teaching future is under a cloud. A very dark cloud.

Chapter Twenty-Four

Keeping the Wolf from the Door

How have I coped all of these years? How have I been keeping my spirit strong at this time of uncertainty? Whilst medications have given me the quality of life to contribute in the world, I have needed much more to help me improve my health status. My current situation has reinforced the importance of simply doing all of the things that I love, if and when, I am able. It is so important, whether it be watching movies, reading books, listening to music or podcasts, watching the footy or getting into the garden – anything that brings me peace and happiness. Spending more time with my family and friends has been imperative in being able to stay positive and less isolated. The support from loved ones is essential in being able to ask for help when I need it and knowing that help will be there. Just as importantly is knowing that it's okay to drift away from family members, friends or work colleagues who are not giving me the love and support I need. If they are causing me stress due to their selfishness or insensitivity, then I will not hesitate to pull back or walk away from those relationships. I will always put myself first. This has been helpful throughout my Lupus Warrior life and more crucial than ever at this moment.

Whilst being a somewhat 30-year veteran of lupus, I don't wish to appear as arrogant in my advice or recommendations for what has worked for me in managing my lupus. I would never assume that what is working for me will work for someone else with lupus. But if I may, I would like to share with fellow Lupus Warriors and readers alike how I am trying to cope each day and what I have found comfort in being able to do, in staying as well as possible with lupus.

In the past, I have attended general yoga, Body Balance and tai chi classes, but intermittently. The state of my lupus and the stress of teaching have impacted on how regularly I have been able to attend these classes. However, during the last few years, particularly since my fibromyalgia diagnosis, I have been more dedicated to my physical health, attending regular classes of Dru Yoga. These classes also include relaxation and meditation practices. Dru Yoga, quite simply, has changed my life. Our teacher, Michelle, is amazing. In addition to her Dru Yoga teaching, she is currently studying to become a qualified osteopath. Her understanding of the human body is constantly evolving as her osteopathy studies help to direct even greater insight into her yoga teaching. Michelle is extremely gifted in her yoga practice, combining beautiful, uplifting mantras and meditations with specific movement and postures. I leave each of her classes in deep reflection, as gratitude to be alive, to be moving my body, to be well enough to be able to nurture myself in this way, lifts me up with greater hope and purpose. I feel so fortunate to be one of Michelle's students.

I have become muscularly stronger and more relaxed as a result of these classes. Over time and with dedicated practice, I have felt my muscles lengthen. The stiffness in my joints welcomes the gentle movements that make up this type of yoga practice. At times, yoga can be painful and challenging but I don't push through when I realise my limits. It feels so great to be able to keep moving and trying to keep my body as strong and as flexible as possible. Even when I am feeling average, once I have started moving and stretching, my body is grateful. Focusing on my breathing is so important too. I have learnt to stop regularly during each day and regulate my breathing. I have a conversation with myself and assess areas of tension I have in my body, which helps me to understand how I am feeling each day and how much rest I need.

Aside from Dru Yoga postures, Michelle is teaching us the importance of relaxation. At least ten-to-twenty minutes of practising relaxation techniques a day is imperative in the body's ability to slow down and let go of daily stress that we may be holding. Battling chronic pain creates much stress in the body. I am finding it extremely beneficial to spend time each day trying to relax and let go. By contracting my major muscle groups whilst lying down and using breathing techniques to focus on such contractions, it is helping me to find a stillness within any pain I am experiencing. By trying to let go of any tightness in my body, I am also helping my body to release stored toxins and as much inflammation as possible. Restorative yoga postures are also helpful in relaxation and regulating my breathing.

I've become extremely dedicated to this yoga practice. I look at my body with more respect and gratitude, with more care and love. I am disappointed if I am unwell and unable to make it to yoga class. It has become a mandatory component of my approach to managing life with lupus. It is just as important as taking my medication.

In addition to attending Dru Yoga classes, I have been beginning each day with a five-minute Dru Yoga prana called Prana Kriyas. It is a beautiful sequence of gentle stretches that is so helpful to wake me up and get me moving for the day. Additionally, I have started to do short meditations to help me focus on my spirit. I am trying, and I stress the word trying, to complete these practices every day when I wake up. I find that these practices help me to direct myself forward into the day with a greater awareness of what I feel I am capable of achieving that day. If I am really tired and struggling, this conversation helps me to be kinder to myself; to not fight the fatigue and pain but to accept it and let go. I have found over the years that it is detrimental to my lupus, and to myself, to push through and fight my pain and fatigue. Inevitably, it will make me sicker. Acceptance of being unwell becomes easier when I simply reassure myself that I am doing my best and that anything I am able to do for that day is a gift in itself.

If you are a Lupus Warrior and are unable to attend yoga classes, there are some wonderful clips on YouTube that can help you practice yoga at home. There are so many you can peruse through and find something that suits your abilities. I encourage you to try if you haven't already. It may change your life too!

Having regular relaxation and stone massages has also helped in easing my pain, whenever I have been unwell. The heat from the stone massage is so healing, particularly when my muscles and joints are feeling so sore and painful. Being in so much pain makes the body so uptight and stressed. For me, it feels so soothing to pay attention to all of those little niggles! Massage is also a great way of eliminating the body of all of the toxins that build up from my medications. It's an expensive practice and I don't get to have them as often as I'd like, but I make it a priority because I believe it's so beneficial for me. Regular warm baths at home are also extremely helpful. Adding Epsom salts to the water to help ease the muscle aches and pains can be very effective and another strategy in trying to stay more relaxed.

Lighting a candle every single night is extremely helpful for my ability to wind down from the day. It may not sound like a big deal, but it really helps me to shut out my problems. I find it really comforting. It's a reflection of my yoga practices too, as the scents they produce are very soothing. Vanilla candles are my favourite. Switching off all of the lights and watching the flicker of that candle flame helps me to feel calmer, still and quiet. I'm sure every single Lupus Warrior has a special practice or practices that help them to manage each day. I have no doubt this would be one of them. I aim to buy and practice using essential oils more regularly for their lovely calming and medicinal properties too.

* * *

It's so important for people with lupus to keep moving. However, battling the constant fatigue of lupus challenges me and many Lupus Warriors in being able to complete regular physical activity, therefore making it hard to achieve my goal of going for regular walks. Completing my Dru Yoga classes is a huge achievement for me, so to add regular walks into my routine can be challenging. I won't push myself to go for a walk if I don't feel well. It's tough for Lupus Warriors to exercise regularly, particularly when you are working and are exhausted at the end of each day. Picking the safest time of the day, away from those dangerous sun and UV rays also makes it a challenge. To avoid these rays, I must get up super early and that is hard, as I just want to get as much rest as possible. Walking in the evening is the only other suitable time, but it too, presents its challenges. Day light saving time helps but winter and colder, dark days reduce the window of time to walk safely in the evenings. Whilst it is hard to sustain regular walking routines, it is one of my most important goals, and having goals is so important in reaching forward when you have lupus.

* * *

Paying more attention to my diet has also been very beneficial in trying to return to the best of health, which is possible for me. I've been seeing an excellent dietitian, Nathalie, who has encouraged me to eat more fibre-enriched foods and more fruits and vegetables each day. I have tried to be more adventurous and eat a wider range of fruits and vegetables, specifically those with as many different colours, pigments and nutrients as possible. The aim is to reduce inflammation in my body and to also have the best gut health possible, which is crucial in helping to control lupus. These foods help the body to do that.

Remarkably, as a result of eating more fruit, vegetables and natural grains, some of my blood tests have shown slight improvement in the reduction of inflammation in my body, which is such a positive and encouraging result. My dietitian has also taught me to monitor the portions of protein-enriched foods I've been eating to ensure that I am not eating too much protein. This may help to control my problem of having traces of protein active in my urine.

In researching suitable recipes and foods that fight inflammation in the body, it has concerned me to discover that there are a few books and websites available that promote the idea that by eating specific foods or a specific diet, lupus can go into complete remission. I am very troubled by this as these ideas are being promoted by qualified dietitians and nutritionists. Please know, particularly if you are a Lupus Warrior, that currently there is no cure for lupus and that, more importantly, there is no 'lupus diet' that you can follow that will make your lupus symptoms disappear or go into remission. Such publications are incredibly misleading and dangerous. You must keep taking your medication and follow your rheumatologist's instructions.

Whilst following a diet high in foods with anti-inflammatory properties can reduce inflammation in the body, there is no scientific proof that following a lupus diet, will ease your symptoms. I have read heartbreaking stories where those with lupus have stopped taking their medication and, over time, have tragically died. Lupus is a serious disease and must be respected. So, I urge my fellow Lupus Warriors to stay medicated, follow your rheumatologist's instructions and to eat a diet low in processed foods but rich in whole foods, fresh fruit and vegetables.

* * *

In addition to eating a diet of more natural, raw, wholesome foods, coffee has continued to be a source of joy for me and a compulsory component of my mornings each day. I love a good latte! It really helps lift me at the start of each day. I suffer from low blood pressure, which can leave me feeling extremely breathless. The caffeine buzz it gives me helps to get my heart beating a little faster. In turn, helping to increase my blood pressure and improve my breathing. Additionally, my rheumatologist gave me the best medical advice I have ever received. She had come to learn that on the day each week that I have my methotrexate, an increase in caffeine via a latte or two, helps my body to absorb the methotrexate more effectively. So, medically, it is extremely beneficial for me too. Win-win! *Woo–hoo!*

Visiting my local cafés for a coffee, is also one of my favourite things to do. I love to sit and 'smell the roses'. I love to watch the world go by. Seeing people enjoying time with their loved ones is heartening and uplifting. A sense of community is strengthened too, as I get to know the baristas and waitstaff over time. It's also a great feeling to arrive at a café for coffee after spending weeks isolated and in bed during a lupus flare. My senses are ignited when I take that first sip; my cup of joy, my cup of courage. In these moments, I reflect very deeply about being on the other side of a flare and knowing how lucky I am to feel better, out of bed and back into the world again. I cherish that feeling. It's the best.

* * *

Aside from all of these practices, at times when I am struggling and feeling overwhelmed, I take much comfort in reading the stories of fellow Lupus Warriors. I don't necessarily need to speak to anyone with lupus. I just feel less alone, particularly when I read of the amazing journeys and experiences they have had. They make me appreciate my life even more. I have attended numerous lupus conferences over the years, symposiums where medical progress in developing lupus treatments is discussed by rheumatologists and research scientists. Unfortunately, at these gatherings, there can be limited opportunity to meet fellow Lupus Warriors as you are listening to so many presenters. However, seeing the range of people in attendance, the demographic and representation of those with lupus, gives me strength that I am not alone. I have attended a couple of lupus support groups during the earlier years of having lupus but found that they were not quite for me. It felt for me to be a very competitive environment in regard to who was 'the sickest'. I don't need to diminish my battle by comparing my pain to the pain of others.

However, maybe these groups just weren't the right fit for me. My quiet, shy nature is likely to be the problem too! Support groups offer much solace for those with lupus, as you are in the company of people who truly understand what you are experiencing. But for me, sometimes I need a break from thinking or talking about lupus. I already live with it every day.

In addition to the stories of Lupus Warriors, I find even more inspiration from reading the stories of other people with chronic illnesses, whether it be someone with multiple sclerosis or rheumatoid arthritis. Being able to put myself in the shoes of other chronic illness sufferers, particularly those with autoimmune diseases, helps me to focus on what I *can* do, not what I *can't* do. It widens my awareness and understanding of how people with chronic illness cope in the wider world. They don't know it, but they inspire me and give me strength. They give me hope.

* * *

Ultimately, I have found that having goals such as attending Dru yoga classes, regularly walking, eating and sleeping well, are integral to maintaining a hopeful, positive attitude each day. For me, I always need something to reach for – to give me purpose. Being sick is already out of my control, so trying to find realistic, achievable ways of moving forward in the form of these types of goals helps me to recognise and appreciate the progress I am making, no matter how big or small.

When I am having a lupus flare and unable to go to yoga or continue my walks, it can feel frustrating, particularly when I have been able to do these things regularly and with much strength and rigour. However, because I have found a way over time to incorporate these practices into my life, I have built space for myself to be able to return to these goals after bouts of illness. And that makes me feel good, as I have something to look forward to each day that I know is making a difference in how I approach life with lupus. It helps to keep the wolf from my door.

Epilogue

How do I keep moving forward at this time of uncertainty? I wish to return to teaching, but I am recognising that my life as a teacher has changed and no matter how positive I am about being well enough to return to teaching in the future, I know in my heart that I cannot manage this workload anymore. If I return to the classroom, I may last for a little while, but I will inevitably continue to plunge deeper and deeper into more lupus flares – flares that are likely to be harder to climb back from in addition to my battle with fibromyalgia and an ageing, lupus-affected body. Students, particularly during adolescence and young adulthood, need teachers that they can rely on. And disappointingly, over time, I became a teacher that my students were unable to rely on, no matter how hard I tried.

Upon much reflection, it has been a long time coming. Secondary teaching has become an extremely tough job. As stated previously, I have watched many healthy, vibrant teachers leave the profession in recent years. Burnt out, disillusioned and dejected, as their hard work and efforts have not been completely valued by their students, parents or employers, as they have deserved to be. Society has changed since I began teaching and I, too, have felt disappointed with the increased lack of respect for teachers and the sacrifices we make in order to give our students our very best in helping them to achieve academic success. The hours and hours of unpaid work have continued to climb during my twenty years of teaching, even more so since the introduction of laptop computers into the classroom. We have become more accessible via email by colleagues, students and parents – 24/7. Hundreds and hundreds of people in the school community are able to question you, judge you and simply add to your already expanded workload, at any time of the day.

Over time, I noticed my energy and goodwill starting to fracture when senior students began questioning the way I had assessed their work. For example, a score of 26 out of 30 was suddenly not seen as an excellent achievement anymore. In recent times, students began to challenge my judgement and beg for re-assessment in order to find scrappy half marks here and there, in the hope of increasing their scores back up to a possible 30 out of 30. It is exhausting, as both a teacher and an adult, to have a seventeen-year-old student stand in front of you, challenging the way you have assessed their work. The lack of respect is jarring let alone confronting. Their combativeness is at times threatening and forceful too, as they demand to receive what they feel are the marks they believe they are entitled to.

This generation has been empowered to believe that they have the right to challenge authority. Whilst there are positives to be gained in having a new generation that is more socially aware, seeing this self-righteous behaviour in action has progressively challenged my love for teaching. The exhaustion of having to defend or explain my actions, when really, I shouldn't have to but need to because some students simply don't understand what they have done wrong. Trying to instil a lifetime of good manners that have been missing from their young lives is also exasperating, not to mention the frustration of having to waste valuable class time to discipline students at the age of eighteen, who are legally adults and are clearly not committed to their studies, at the expense of a respectful, peaceful learning environment for students who do want to learn. More shockingly is seeing parents support their child's disruptive behaviour, defending at times indefensible behaviours. I never anticipated the day in my teaching career that I would be the person ridiculed by a parent or a student because the student hadn't completed a task I had clearly set. Isn't it meant to be the other way around?

When I reflect on how challenging teaching has become, and how difficult I have found it to overcome these disheartening moments, I recall a cataclysmic day in 2012 when I was knocked to the ground during a school yard fight whilst I was on yard duty. A turf war between some Year 11 and Year 12 boys had been brewing in the school yard for weeks. My warnings of impending trouble to Year Level coordinators fell on deaf ears. I remember saying at the time, just how unsafe I felt on yard duty. I recall joking that I felt I needed a baton and capsicum spray every time I took my post. For these weren't boys anymore. Aged between sixteen and eighteen, they were young men. And their physical presence in the school yard, standing together in a group, was extremely imposing and threatening.

Inevitably, the impending fight broke out. Prior to this violent outbreak, I had sensed tensions brewing. Suddenly, a group of these students began throwing food at each other. Another teacher and I tried talking calmly to the two main culprits, hoping to stop their aggression from escalating even further than it already had. In doing so, whilst trying to move these students away from the crowd of other students, these two students started to mouth off at one another. Their verbal exchange quickly became physical, as they started pushing each other. A student, from the now large group of students watching these boys sparring with one another, leapt from his nearby seat and charged at one of these boys. From then on, other boys watching from the crowd bolted from their seats and joined in by jumping on top of the boys who were fighting with one another. They were like animals – lunging, clawing and punching each other.

Pleas for these boys to stop went unheard. What occurred next happened so quickly that I couldn't get out of the way in time. In the hectic affray of punching one another, one of the students fell on top of me and I crashed straight to the ground. He would have been over 6 feet tall, broad-shouldered and simply too huge for my comparatively slight frame. The boys, thankfully, stopped fighting as soon as they saw that I had been knocked to the ground. CCTV footage in the school yard would later show that I was standing there one minute, and suddenly, gone the next.

Epilogue

Lying on the cold concrete, I had somehow managed to protect my fall by folding myself into the foetal position as I fell to the ground. This instinct to protect myself saved me from harm. Amazingly, I didn't hit my head on the concrete or break any bones. But I felt extremely sore and confused. I was shaking. Aside from feeling shocked at what I had just experienced, even more surprising was the sickening sound of a student mocking me in front of the now large crowd of students, who had gathered to see what had happened. 'Oh my God. Look at her. She's crying!' I lifted my head and suddenly realised that I had tears streaming down my face.

I've never forgotten the sound of his voice, his cruel words, as he mocked me for going into shock. A physical shock I had no control over. The lilt of both joy and surprise in his voice, of seeing a teacher hurt and upset. Defenceless. His callous ridicule of me was then quashed by the sound of subsequent laughter from fellow students at hearing his cry, as they, too, enjoyed the spectacle of seeing me strewn onto the ground – fragile and vulnerable. These were students I didn't know, and who didn't know me, that is until I spotted one of my Year 12 students in the crowd, as she too, joined in the jeering and seeming amusement of my fall. Seeing her participate in this cruel, heartless behaviour was devastating. I had a positive relationship with this student, so to see her react to my plight in this way was truly shocking. Maybe it was the power of being amongst her peer group – that pressure to behave like them. I will never know. To this day, I wish I hadn't spotted her in the crowd. It was so much to overcome when I returned to the classroom later on, knowing that every time I had to teach her, I was reminded of her choice to belittle me in a moment where I needed her care and compassion.

Not one student came to my aid that day. Feeling humiliated and simply shattered, I found the strength to slowly stand up. Without making eye contact with any of these students, I'm sure I cut a forlorn figure as I walked gingerly to my office. To safety.

Hours after my fall, as I sat in the toilet of my local GP, attending the compulsory health and safety doctor's visit after a workplace incident, peeing into a cup to check for internal bleeding, the shock at what I had just experienced began to churn inside my heart and mind. What had happened? This was a day at school. A day in my workplace, one where I would return home in a more distressed way than I could imagine. Days before, I received the best news from my rheumatologist: that my lupus was under control. I was in the best health I had been in a long time. I had previously spent months and months tapering off large doses of methotrexate and steroids, slowly climbing ladders, up each row of that Snakes and Ladders board. And I was on my way to making it back to the top. I began to fear that my lupus would flare again as a result of the shock and stress of this fall. Unfortunately, it did.

Within forty-eight hours of this fall, I slipped into another difficult lupus flare. More time absent from work. More absences from my Year 12 classes. More medicine. My rage was palpable. Forget about sliding down the length of a long snake on that pesky game board. The wolf had found me. It not only emerged from what I thought, was its tightly contained box, it not only knocked on my door – it kicked it down. It snarled at me with all of its sharp edges. It roared at me, taunting me to try and fight back, despite knowing that I was at my weakest. And so, I roared back, with tears and anger; defiant, exasperated and then ultimately, distraught, that this merciless wolf, had returned so quickly, despite doing everything I could to keep it in its place.

The depths of my anger terrified me. I had never felt such rage before. And the fact that it took me four long weeks of fighting Senior School to discipline these students accordingly for what had happened to me was the final straw. Resentful and dejected, it took all of my strength and what hope I had left to climb my way out of this dark place I had somehow come to land in. I was curled up, hurt and wounded at the bottom of that wretched Snakes and Ladders board, praying that I could roll the dice and find my way forward again.

* * *

In the months and years that followed this fall, having lupus and then fibromyalgia became an even greater, unrelenting struggle. I felt myself slowly diminishing in strength and spirit. Teaching was also upping the ante, demanding me to be tougher, stronger and more forgiving than I was well enough to be. When I transport myself back to that moment, lying on that cold concrete, shocked and alone, I have no doubt my love of teaching changed irrevocably that day. It was the precipice for the eventual slow decline in my health that has continued ever since.

How does the realisation that I'm unlikely to return to regular classroom teaching make me feel? I am heartbroken. Sad. I miss seeing the smiling faces of my students, of watching them grow and shine over time as

Epilogue

they discover joy and pride in their achievements. I miss the laughter, the banter and joy of their company. And I miss those moments when I am feeling truly well – organised, strong in voice, clear in mind and in full flight, imparting a new idea, a new way of thinking and simply connecting with my students. Teaching – it is the greatest feeling, knowing that I am trying my very best to hopefully make a difference in their lives.

However, it is the inevitable realisation that I no longer have the stoicism or resilience to overcome the insurmountable, relentless stress secondary school teaching has become. Whilst I do not wish to rule out teaching in the future or extinguish that hope from my life, I know in my heart, that I need to be sensible and realistic about my choices. I must remember that Lupus Warriors need to play the long game. As a Lupus Warrior, I need to play smart. And with that, the long game needs to play fair. Secondary school teaching isn't playing fair anymore.

So, I am on another journey of acceptance. In all of the teachings that having lupus brings, I know I must put into practice what I have learnt in being able to let go and to embrace the unknown. In doing this, I must remember how amazing it has been that I have even been able to teach. I need to focus on all of the blessings of being able to fulfil my dream. But I am scared. I feared that this day would come. I just didn't want it to. I hoped it wouldn't be this soon. I hoped it wouldn't be this way.

My rheumatologist, Michelle, says that I have the body of a ninety-year-old. That puts everything into perspective for me. For having lupus and fibromyalgia have most certainly defined me. I read so many stories where those with illness shout loudly, 'But I won't let lupus define me!' This leaves me confused, because from where I sit, lupus has defined every inch of who I am. It has given me greater empathy and compassion for those who are battling chronic diseases or challenging health issues. I am a kinder, more considerate and less judgmental person because of lupus. I am more patient and adaptable when faced with new challenges, because I have learned to surrender. I have accepted that I am suffering from (at present) a chronic, incurable disease. It has defined very clear boundaries for many of my capabilities in getting through daily life. If I don't respect those limitations, I am at risk of overdoing it and harming my health and myself in the process. It means that I have not accepted my diagnosis – that I am not at peace with having lupus.

I don't wish to live in a state of defiance. I do not wish to rise up against an enemy I cannot defeat. I don't want to be embittered or angry about the lemons that have been given to me, for maybe, they are not lemons after all. What energy I do have is precious, and I must use it wisely. What I must do is simply co-exist with lupus, this vicious wolf, and keep persevering as best I can – to be smart enough to know that lupus is the boss. That's all I can do, for I am not in control of what it can do. I can take my pills, de-stress and be as spiritually and physically strong as I can possibly be, but at this moment, the wolf is top dog and it is not leaving me anytime soon.

Currently, there has only been one new drug specifically developed for lupus over the last fifty years. In my mind, with so many Lupus Warriors throughout the world, this is infuriating. Why this insidious, debilitating and life-threatening disease has been ignored for so many years is a complete mystery to me. But it occurred to me one day. I asked myself, 'Rachel, what have you done during these thirty years of having lupus to create more change and awareness of lupus? Just waited for a cure?' Well, the answer is yes. Yes, I have. I have also been waiting for change. Waiting for the world to know what lupus is so that I don't have to keep explaining it. Waiting for different, more effective and less toxic, side-effect-inducing medicine to treat and possibly cure my symptoms.

Change only happens with greater education and awareness. So, writing this book is my best effort in being able to contribute to this change. I, too, am responsible for how lupus awareness must change. How can I expect people to know what lupus is, if I haven't tried hard enough to play my part and make sense of my lupus battle and share it with them? Despite my quiet, shy persona, I must keep overcoming the discomfort I feel when sharing my story as a thirty-year Lupus Warrior. I must hope, like I do when I read about the lives of others with lupus or other chronic illnesses, that fellow Lupus Warriors can feel less alone in their battle when they read my story. Just as important, hopefully I can educate those who are unfamiliar with lupus and who can, in turn, affect more change by being able to continue educating others of the perplexities and seriousness of this disease.

***

So, what now? How do I keep making lemonade in my life? Well, all I have at the moment is each day – like every single person in the world. I am trying hard not to look too far ahead but it is hard when friends and family ask me what I am going to do. Making each day count by truly letting go of as much of my stress and worry as possible is my priority, so that I can reduce as much lupus inflammation in my body as possible and return to being as well as I can be. I know I must keep my heart wide open, to trust that I am exactly where I am meant to be. That everything is as it should be. To help me embrace this state of being, I must find courage. I must choose happiness. And I must live bravely. To just live. But it isn't easy, for being hopeful and brave takes much reflection, much energy and much effort. Not knowing what my working future will look like and worrying about how I am going to take care of myself is stressful too – an ongoing challenge in following my mantra of staying positive.

For many years, I have framed an acronym for the word lupus. It is a positive spin on this word, to help me feel brighter. It sits in my study and reads as follows:

Lupus = Lift Up, Persevere, Use Strength

And so, that is what I must do. To simply lift up and keep persevering with strength in all I am able to do. To embody the sentiments of what the word lupus can stand for, not what it is or what it does. To believe in my heart that I will be okay. To keep trying and doing my best to keep the wolf quiet, contained deep inside that box, tucked away – lid shut tightly.

Acknowledgements

I acknowledge the traditional owners of this country, specifically, I pay my respects and gratitude to the traditional custodians of the land I live on, the Wurundjeri willam people.

To my publisher, Blaise van Hecke – I am so glad I found some courage and walked through your door at Busybird Publishing. Your warmth, encouragement and support for my idea has strengthened my self-belief that I could write this book. Thank you for calmly guiding me through every step of this process.

Thank you, Josephine Hong, for your outstanding, thorough and fastidious contributions to editing my manuscript. I've learnt so much from the editing process we have shared together. Thank you so much for your patience and guidance.

'Thank you to the Busybird publishing team, particularly Kev Howlett and Les Zigomanis, for designing and producing my book. I am beyond grateful.

To the amazing James Fosdike – you have created an extraordinary illustration, capturing my true spirit as a Lupus Warrior in a most striking portrait. Your work here is truly beautiful and I am extremely grateful for your contribution to my book – thank you so much.

Acknowledgements

Thank you to my Disability Liaison Officer Margaret McKeough at Deakin, for guiding me through university, ensuring my special needs were met with respect and without prejudice by my lecturers and tutors. Thank you to Jackie Dean for being my advocate during my senior years at secondary school.

To the many general practitioners, specialists and nurses who have cared for me during my time of ill health over 30 years – thank you.

To my rheumatologist Dr Michelle Tellus – thank you for your respect and humanity in being the first specialist to see and treat me as a whole person. Your determination, dedication and care in your endeavour to always find the best, most practical solutions in treating my lupus is incomparable – thank you.

To my GP Dr Joanne McClean – thank you for over 27 years of care, support and good humour, particularly 13 years of weekly visits for treatment. To the team at Sherbourne Road Medical Clinic, thank you for always making me feel so cared for and valued.

To my ophthalmologist Dr Peter Meagher and his assistant Vivien for your support and treatment – nearly 30 years of eye check-ups (surely, we have broken a record?!)

To my endocrinologist, Dr Felicity Pyrlis – thank you for your kindness and persistence in trying to find solutions to a very complicated health issue. Your understanding and knowledge of lupus has been nothing short of impressive and a comfort to me during this time of uncertainty with my health – thank you for your support.

To my current and former podiatrists, Sophie Duguid and Sarah Campbell – thank you for being so caring regarding my lupus and for taking good care of my footsies and lightening my step!

To my dietitian, Nathalie Cook – thank you for your support and guidance in helping me to find more effective pathways of nutritious eating. I've learnt so much about the role of inflammation and the gut in treating lupus. Your passion for nutritious, sensible eating and expertise has been instrumental in helping me to achieve improved health. I'm so grateful – thank you for your constant positivity and encouragement.

To the gorgeous girls at Dru Yoga classes – Saturday mornings are brighter with you in them. Thank you, Marg, Judith and Marcia, for your support, interest and encouragement, particularly during the writing of this book.

To my Dru Yoga teacher and friend, Michelle Harris – finding your classes all those years ago has been life-changing. You are such a blessing in my life, for you have helped me to nurture and cultivate a disciplined but gentle, consistent yoga practice in my life that has generated much healing in my physical and spiritual health. You are an inspiration – thank you.

To Sonia and the team at Rhodes Hair and Spa, Hawthorn for always nurturing me with beautiful massages, hair treatments and coffee. You make such a difference in lifting me up (not to mention, putting me back together so that I can be presentable in the world again!)

Special thank yous to the staff at all of the cafés I frequent (you know who you are!) Thank you for lifting my spirits with your gifts of the most delicious coffees and meals. Thank you for your interest, encouragement and support during the completion of this book.

To my former primary and secondary school teachers, Andrew Guthrie (formerly Merryweather), Garry Chapman, Jayne Walsh and Kerryn Low. Your dedication, diligence and good humour as fun, caring, supportive teachers helped me to see that teaching is a true vocation and that if I believed in myself and worked hard, I was capable of being a teacher myself. Thank you!

To my former students – please know that being your teacher has been a most honourable experience in my life. Your achievements are my achievements and it has been a privilege to know you and be part of your life's journey. I hope this book is an example of the many messages I would babble on about in class, particularly the message of staying true to yourself and to always persevere and believe in yourself, for anything is possible with pride and hope in your heart.

To former teaching colleagues and friends at Lalor North Secondary College, Sunbury College, Viewbank College and St Helena Secondary College; battling at times a seemingly invisible chronic illness in lupus, I was always very moved to simply be thought of, particularly during the busyness of the school day. Thank you to anyone who gave me a smile, a hug, asked if I was okay or who simply lifted me up with their thoughtfulness, understanding and encouragement.

To my Sunbury friends and former teaching colleagues, Rebecca Kirkham, Shane and Tamara Smith, Peter Freeman and Tholie Forbes, thank you for your friendship, support, professionalism and guidance, which has significantly shaped my teaching practice. Rebecca, thanks for your support and for all of the coffee catch-ups.

Acknowledgements

Greg and Penny Hill, thank you for always caring during many years of friendship. I love our catch-ups and reminiscing about our Viewbank teaching days! Thank you, Ray and Gayle Linsell, for your friendship and support during and after my time at Viewbank. Thank you also to Jenny McKinnis and John Munro for keeping my chin up during challenging times.

To my St Helena friends and former teaching colleagues, Trent Ray, Kay Banes, Liam O'Neill, Sally Hughan and Hannah Vellacott: thank you for your friendship and support over the years. Thank you, Trent, for helping to restore my confidence and belief in myself, particularly during a challenging phase of my teaching career. You are an inspiration. Thank you, Sally, for your friendship and continued support. I'm so grateful for all of the times you stepped into my teaching shoes when I was ill and kept my students on track. Thank you, Kay, for your friendship and wicked sense of humour. You bring joy to everyone you meet. Thank you, Liam, for your like-mindedness and support. Thank you, Hannah, for always lifting me up with your wise and encouraging words.

To Deb Larbey and Michael Boyd – thank you for your friendship and never-ending kindness. You are the best neighbours and friends anyone could hope for! Thank you for always inspiring me to be more caring and charitable through all of the selfless volunteer work you do for cancer awareness and prevention.

To my dear friends, Maree Pell and Chris Hemsworth – I miss you both very much. Both taken way too soon. Your friendship, loving, caring and generous spirits will always live on in my heart xxx

To my Aunty Bron, Uncle Fred and cousins, Martin and Megan – thank you for welcoming me into your family all those years ago and supporting me during my teaching studies. Rest in peace, Fred xx

Karen Bryce, thank you for your example as a caring, dedicated teacher during my high school years. You were instrumental in sparking my own dream to teach. Thank you, Karen, for showing how an act of kindness can help make all the difference in the world during a time of much uncertainty and stress. Driving me home from school all those years ago when I was too ill to walk is still spoken of and appreciated with much affection and gratitude in my family. Thank for you for being my friend.

To Jill Evans – thank you, Jill, for your constant friendship, your thoughtfulness, understanding and for always caring. Your gentle spirit has been a comfort to me during some very difficult times. I treasure our friendship.

To Sue Bamford – thank you, Sue, for your kindness, steadfast friendship and for your encouragement and faith in my ability to persevere in writing this book. Thank you for giving me your time to provide much valued feedback. You are inspiring in every way and I am so blessed to call you my friend.

Jackie Maartensz (nee Orwin), thank you for over 25 years of friendship, love and laughter. Being grouped together at uni to work on our dietitian project at the Royal Children's Hospital in Melbourne all those years ago was quite fortuitous! Thank you for always being so loyal, loving and caring. Thank you to the Maartensz and Orwin families, Darren, Isaac, Leila, Bob and Ange for your love and kindness.

Gypsy, Muffin, Pepe, Milly and Squeak – thank you for all of your cuddles. You were and are the cutest and most loving of all kitty cats xxx

To my brother Ross and sister-in-law Naomi, thank you for your love and support.

Bec, whilst you are my loving sister, you are also my dearest friend. You are the most loving, giving, selfless person I know. Thank you for your generosity, your humour and your support. You are the best. I love you very much, Becsy Girl xxx

Mum and Dad, thank you for your unconditional love, unwavering support, courage and unmatched stoicism. Thank you for always picking me up during the tough times and for helping me to live my life independently and with much dignity. Mum, thank you for all of your thoughtful words of encouragement, guidance, hope and faith. Dad, thank you for always leading by example with your quiet strength, selflessness, modesty and wisdom. I don't know where I'd be without you. I love you both very much xxx

Author's Biography

Rachel Lea has worked as a VCE Health and Human Development and Food Technology teacher for 20 years in the Victorian Government secondary school system. She has had previous written works published in VCE Biology texts and various Deakin University magazines. *Lupus = Lift-Up, Persevere and Use Strength* is her first book. She is currently taking an absence from teaching due to her current health battles. She lives in Melbourne's outer-North with her cute rescue cat, Squeak.

Useful Resources

- Kaleidoscope Fighting Lupus (formerly Molly's fund), American Lupus support foundation, www.kaleidoscopefightinglupus.com
- Lupus Canada, www.lupuscanada.org
- Lupus Foundation of America, www.lupus.org
- Lupus Foundation of NSW, www.lupusnsw.org.au
- Mayo Clinic, www.mayoclinic.org
- Wallace, D.J., *The Lupus Book*, 2019, 6th edition, New York, Oxford University Press

Lupus Support Services

Listed below, are the websites of major lupus support services you can visit for more information about lupus as a disease and also for greater emotional support if you are a Lupus Warrior or carer. They are categorised according to location, with Australian and New Zealand support services listed first:

Lupus Associations in Australia and New Zealand

Victoria

Lupus Victoria

https://www.lupusvictoria.com/blog

https://m.facebook.com/lupusvictoria/

Musculoskeletal Australia

https://www.msk.org.au

New South Wales

Lupus NSW
https://lupusnsw.org.au

Western Australia

Lupus WA
https://www.lupuswa.com.au/lupus-support/

Tasmania

Lupus Tasmania
https://www.lupustasmania.org.au

New Zealand

Arthritis New Zealand
https://www.arthritis.org.nz

International

World Lupus Federation
https://worldlupusfederation.org

USA

Lupus Foundation of America
https://www.lupus.org

Kaleidoscope Fighting Lupus (formerly known as Molly's Fund)
https://kaleidoscopefightinglupus.org

Lupus Corner
 https://lupuscorner.com

Lupus Lyfe
 http://lupuslyfe.com

Canada

Canada
 Lupus Canada
 https://www.lupuscanada.org

UK

Lupus UK
 https://www.lupusuk.org.uk

Lupus Group Ireland
 http://www.lupusgroupireland.com/news.html

Europe

Lupus Europe
 www.lupus-europe.org

Endnotes

1. Mayo Clinic, 2018, 'Chronic Fatigue Syndrome', https://www.mayoclinic.org/diseases-conditions/chronic-fatigue-syndrome/symptoms-causes/syc-20360490
2. Wallace, D.J., *The Lupus* Book, 2019, 6th edition, New York, Oxford University Press
3. Lupus Foundation of America, 2017, 'Lupus symptoms', https://www.lupus.org/resources/common-symptoms-of-lupus
4. Lupus Foundation of America, 'Diagnosing lupus', https://www.lupus.org/resources/diagnosing-lupus-guide
5. Lupus Foundation of America, 2013, 'What is lupus?', https://www.lupus.org/resources/what-is-lupus?utm_campaign=Take_Charge&utm_content
6. Kaleidoscope Fighting Lupus, 'Quick Lupus Facts', https://kaleidoscopefightinglupus.org/about-lupus/what-is-lupus/
7. Australasian Society of Clinical Immunology and Allergy, 2019, 'Systemic Lupus Erythematosus (SLE)', https://www.allergy.org.au/patients/autoimmunity/systemic-lupus-erythematosus-sle
8. Lupus Canada, https://www.lupuscanada.org
9. Lupus Association of NSW, 'What is Lupus?', https://lupusnsw.org.au/understanding-lupus/what-is-lupus/
10. Kaleidoscope Fighting Lupus, 'Systemic Lupus Erythematosus', https://kaleidoscopefightinglupus.org/systemic-lupus-erythematosus-sle/
11. Lupus Foundation of America, 2013, 'Finding the Treatment Approach for You', https://www.lupus.org/resources/finding-the-treatment-approach-for-you
12. Lupus Canada, 'Living With Lupus Q&A', https://www.lupuscanada.org/lupus-questions/
13. Lupus Foundation of America, 2013, 'Prognosis and life expectancy', https://www.lupus.org/resources/prognosis-and-life-expectancy
14. Lupus Foundation of America, 'Lupus facts and statistics', https://www.lupuscanada.org/lupus-questions/
15. Mayo Clinic, 2019, 'Cushing syndrome', https://www.mayoclinic.org/diseases-conditions/cushing-syndrome/symptoms-causes/syc-20351310
16. Mayo Clinic, 2017, 'Raynaud's disease', https://www.mayoclinic.org/diseases-conditions/raynauds-disease/symptoms-causes/syc-20363571
17. Lupus Foundation of America, 'UV exposure: What you need to know', https://www.lupus.org/resources/uv-exposure-what-you-need-to-know
18. National Fibromyalgia Association, 'Fibromyalgia Symptoms', https://fmaware.net/fibromyalgia-symptoms/
19. WebMD, 2019, 'What Is Fibromyalgia?', https://www.webmd.com/fibromyalgia/guide/what-is-fibromyalgia#1
20. Kaleidoscope Fighting Lupus, 'Fibromyalgia and Lupus', https://kaleidoscopefightinglupus.org/fibromyalgia-and-lupus/#1

www.ingramcontent.com/pod-product-compliance
Lightning Source LLC
Chambersburg PA
CBHW071729080526
44588CB00013B/1959